An Introduction to Stata for Health Researchers

An Introduction to Stata for Health Researchers

SVEND JUUL
Institute of Public Health
Department of Epidemiology
Aarhus University
Aarhus, Denmark

A Stata Press Publication
StataCorp LP
College Station, Texas

Stata Press, 4905 Lakeway Drive, College Station, Texas 77845

Contents

Figures

Preface

The main intent behind this book is *empowerment*: I want to help you to benefit from using Stata in your own research. Your research is probably demanding enough as it is, but to many researchers, the technicalities of data management and analysis can cause major problems—sometimes overwhelming problems. Stata has the tools you need; the purpose of this book is to help you use them.

Stata is a versatile program aimed at data management, statistical analysis, and graphics for research. It is dynamic, too, with new and improved tools being added by Stata monthly, and with contributions from an enthusiastic user community daily. This rapid development pace may make the inexperienced user feel a bit lost in what may initially look like a huge jungle. I want to help you become familiar with the basics and to benefit from some of the more advanced analytic tools. I will not be able to demonstrate everything Stata can do, but I hope to help you get started—and more.

This book is an introduction, written for the newcomer who has little or no experience with Stata. But it will also be a valuable companion for more advanced users. Although I wrote the book to meet the newcomer's needs, I chose to build it systematically, e.g., by putting everything about calculations in one chapter, from the basics to the more complex stuff. This systematic structure makes it easy to locate the information you need. Some of the exercises are aimed at beginners.

The systematic approach also means that you should not try to understand or learn everything in the sequence it is presented, e.g., in chapter 4 on command syntax. But now that you know it is there, when you have a general question on Stata's grammar, you can look in that chapter to find the answer.

The book's primary audience is people working with health research. When selecting which data management and analysis tools to demonstrate, I chose the tools that in my experience are most often used in health research. But there is much more to it than what is shown in this book. Official Stata has hundreds of commands; I selected a few of them and point to some other commands that might be useful to you. In addition to the official Stata commands, there are a thousand user-generated contributions. I point to a few of them, too, and demonstrate how to find and use them.

Writing this book has been a joy (mostly). One of the best parts of the experience has been the enthusiastic discussions I have had with people at StataCorp. In particular, Alan Riley, Vince Wiggins, and Bennet Fauber have given a lot of useful input, and Terri Schroeder and Lisa Gilmore have skillfully prepared the manuscript for printing. The most important input, however, was from the students I taught and supervised.

If you believe you have discovered an error, or if you have a suggestion for improving the book, please send an email to ishr@soci.au.dk.

Svend Juul

Aarhus, Denmark
February 2006

Online supplements

This book has several online resources associated with it, which you can find at

http://www.stata-press.com/books/ishr.html

Resources on this web site include

- Datasets.
- Programs, such as those for easy handling of output (see chapter 17).
- A do-file for each graph shown. I sometimes show only the minimal command needed to display a graph; the corresponding do-file includes all options used to obtain the final graph.
- A link to supplementary materials.
- Errors and corrections (if any) will be shown in an *Errata* section. If you believe you have discovered an error, or if you have a suggestion for improving the book, please send an email to ishr@soci.au.dk. Do not use this address to obtain help; for help, see chapter 2.
- There may be other resources placed on the web site after this book goes to press, so visit it to see what else appears there.

Notation in this book

Stata commands and the corresponding output are generally shown in these typefaces:

```
. webuse lowbirth.dta
(Applied Logistic Regression, Hosmer & Lemeshow)

. keep pairid low smoke

. list in 1/4, sepby(pairid)
```

	pairid	low	smoke
1.	1	0	0
2.	1	1	1
3.	2	0	0
4.	2	1	0

The commands you can enter are shown in boldface and are preceded by a period that represents Stata's command prompt. Do not type the period.

When referring to menu items, I use a sans serif font, such as

Statistics ▷ Summaries, tables, & tests ▷ Nonparametric tests of hypotheses

I use slant to show keystrokes, such as *Ctrl-C* and *Enter*.

1 Getting started

This chapter describes how to install, update, and customize Stata and demonstrates the use of the various windows.

Before starting to work with Stata, you must know your operating system and make some decisions on how to use it. Actually, this requirement applies to any software, but it is especially critical when you work with your own data, which may have been collected at great expense. I describe primarily how to work in Windows, and I refer to [GSW] (the *Getting Started with Stata for Windows* manual). However, the other *Getting Started* manuals are organized similarly, and users of other platforms can use the relevant [GS] manual.

First, you must decide where to put your own files, such as datasets and other documents. The newer Windows versions initially suggest that you store them somewhere along a long branch starting with `Documents and Settings`. I recommend that you choose a simpler structure and store your own documents in subfolders under your main personal folder; in this book, we will store files in subfolders of `C:\docs`. For more specific advice on how to work with Windows, see Appendix B.

In the book's examples, I assume that you downloaded the datasets associated with the book to `C:\docs\ishr`, but you can store them where you wish; see http://www.stata-press.com/books/ishr.html for instructions.

Sections 1.6 and 1.9 are exercises. If you are a newcomer to Stata, I recommend that you do the exercises in section 1.6. You might later decide to return to sections 1.7 and 1.8 and the exercises in section 1.9.

1.1 Installing and updating Stata

Installation

Insert the installation CD, and follow the instructions. [GSW] **1 Installation** gives more details, if needed.

Stata suggests that you use `C:\data` as the default working directory. I recommend that you choose `C:\docs` or whatever your personal main folder is; see section 1.3.

Before we get started, you should update Stata.

Updating

It is important that you update Stata before you proceed. StataCorp regularly releases free enhancements and bug fixes to Stata. It is a good idea to make sure that you have the very latest set of changes. To obtain these, you must be connected to the Internet. For more about updating, see [GSW] **19 Using the Internet** and [R] **update**.

From Stata's menu bar, select

> Help ▷ Official updates

A Viewer window opens (see section 1.4), which tells you that the executable (the main program wstata.exe[1]) currently installed is from 17 Dec 2005 and the ado-files are from 20 Dec 2005:

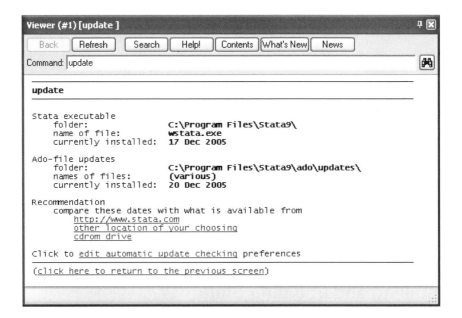

---

1. wstata.exe is the name of the executable for Intercooled Stata. For Stata/SE, it is wsestata.exe, and for Small Stata, it is wsmstata.exe. If you use a Macintosh or Unix computer, the names will differ slightly.

Follow the recommendation, and click the link http://www.stata.com to get the following response:

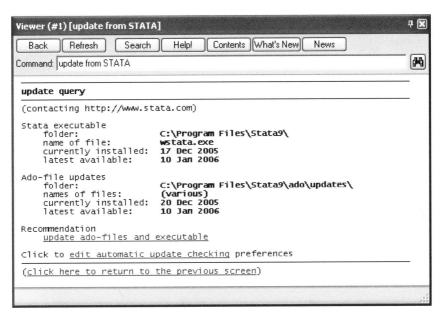

You are told that there is a new executable and ado-file updates from 10 Jan 2006. Follow the recommendation; in this case, click update ado-files and executable. You are now told which ado-files were updated. This time the executable is updated, too (in most updates only ado-files are updated):

(Continued on next page)

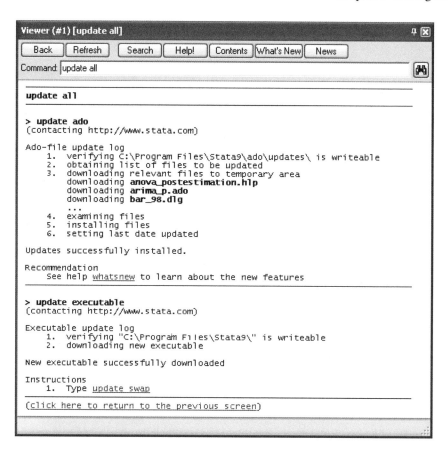

IMPORTANT: If you download a new executable, you must install it before you can use it. Do that by typing the command `update swap` or by clicking the `update swap` link. The screen flickers a bit—and then you have the updated version of Stata. If the message, `no; data in memory would be lost` is displayed, it means that you have a dataset loaded, so you must save your dataset and then `update swap` or, if you do not want to save your data, you may enter the following commands in the Command window:

```
. clear
```

```
. update swap
```

After an update, you can see what was replaced and why, by typing

```
. help whatsnew
```

Downloading the files for an update may take some time, so be patient. If you lose the connection during the update, no harm is done, and you can safely repeat the procedure (and be more patient).

If you have trouble updating, see the FAQs (frequently asked questions; see section 2.3) on updating at http://www.stata.com/support/updates/ for some alternative solutions.

Updating regularly is a must!

Stata will ask you regularly if you want to check for updates. Accept the offer; it is easy—and important.

Where did Stata put the program files?

When installing, Stata typically creates the folders shown below. The main program (the executable) is installed in `C:\Program Files\Stata9`, whereas many commands are defined by ado-files (see section 17.3) to be installed in `C:\Program Files\Stata9\ado\base`. When updating, Stata installs new and revised ado-files in
`C:\Program Files\Stata9\ado\updates`.

Many ado-files have been written by creative users, not by Stata; see section 2.2 to learn how to locate them. Such files are installed in `C:\ado\plus`. You can store your own ado-files in `C:\ado\personal`. The main folders for the Stata program typically are

```
C:\
    ado
        personal          Your own creations (e.g., ado-files, profile.do)
        plus              Downloaded "unofficial" ado-files,
                              e.g., user-written programs
    ...
    Program Files
        Stata9            The main program (the executable)
            ado
                base      Official ado-files as shipped with Stata
                updates   Official ado-file updates
```

You can display these folders by typing the `sysdir` command:

```
. sysdir
    STATA:  C:\Program Files\Stata9\
  UPDATES:  C:\Program Files\Stata9\ado\updates\
     BASE:  C:\Program Files\Stata9\ado\base\
     SITE:  C:\Program Files\Stata9\ado\site\
     PLUS:  c:\ado\plus\
 PERSONAL:  c:\ado\personal\
```

When you issue a command, Stata searches the currently active folder and these folders (called the *ado-path*) in the sequence shown until it finds a command with that name. If the command fails, Stata displays an error message.

1.2   Starting and stopping Stata

Starting Stata

There are several ways to start Stata; see [GSW] **2 Starting and stopping Stata**. In Windows, you can use one of the following methods:

- Select [Start] ▷ Programs ▷ Stata.
- If you have a Stata desktop icon (see section 1.3), double-click it.
- Open Explorer or My Computer, and double-click a file with the extension .do or .dta.

But take care: any of these methods will open a new Stata session, even if one is already active, and you may end up with two or three Stata sessions running at the same time. If that is not what you intended, it is confusing, and you may have problems with your log files (see section 1.7).

Stopping Stata

To stop Stata, you can do one of the following things:

- Select File ▷ Exit.
- Click the ✖ button in the upper-right corner of the screen.
- Enter exit in the Command window.

If you have modified the data in memory without saving the modifications, you will be asked to choose **Save** or **Don't save**. If you make modifications intended to be permanent, make them with a do-file ending with a save command (see section 6.1)—saving the modified dataset with a new name. If you have done that, Stata will not ask the question. If Stata asks you, it is likely that you made modifications not intended to be permanent, and the risk is that you overwrite good data with bad data if you respond **Save**.

You can avoid the above question by entering exit, clear in the Command window; then the current memory contents will not be saved.

1.3   Customizing Stata (Windows)

Important (Windows 98 and ME users only)

These Windows versions have restricted capacity for dialogs. To avoid problems, enter the following in the Command window—just once:

```
. set smalldlg on, permanently
```

The permanently option means that this command will be in effect forever.

Create desktop shortcut icon

If a desktop shortcut icon was not created during installation, use Explorer or My Computer to locate the executable in `C:\Program files\Stata9`. In Intercooled Stata for Windows, it is `wstata.exe`; in Stata/SE, it is `wsestata.exe`. Right-click it, and drag it to the desktop, where you select **Create Shortcut**.

Right-click the new icon and select **Properties**. Select your personal main folder as the start folder; in this book's examples, it is select `C:\docs` (see Appendix B on Windows). Below you will find the reasons for this recommendation:

- You should put your own text, graph, data files, and do-files in folders organized and named by subject, not by the program that created them; otherwise, you will end up confused.

- All of your own folders should be in subfolders under one personal main folder, e.g., `C:\docs`. The two advantages to this are

  - You avoid mixing your own files with program files.
  - You can set up a consistent backup strategy (see section 18.9).

- Above all: do not put your own files in the `C:\Program files\Stata9` folder (the Stata program folder).

1.4   Windows in Stata

[GSW] **4 The Stata user interface** gives a nice introduction to the windows, including the use of the various buttons.

In each window you may right-click; one option is to change font for that type of window; see [GSW] **Setting font and window preferences**. Select a fixed-width font, e.g., Lucida Console 9 pt for the windows displaying output, i.e., the Results and Viewer windows.

Start by maximizing the main Stata window (click the ▣ button; middle button in the upper-right corner). Next adjust the other windows' sizes and locations with the mouse; the windows should look approximately like those in figure 1.1. When finished, make your choices the default by selecting

  Prefs ▷ Manage preferences ▷ Save preferences

Save your preferences with a name, e.g., `myprefs`. If you somehow lost the settings, you can easily recreate them by selecting

  Prefs ▷ Manage preferences ▷ Load preferences

You can control the behavior of the windows by selecting

  Prefs ▷ General Preferences ▷ Windowing

I suggest to check (postponing any experiments to another day) "Disable XP themes" and to uncheck all other options. Look at the possibilities in [GSW] **4 The Stata user interface**. Also find a small movie demonstrating some of the possibilities at http://www.ats.ucla.edu/stat/stata/faq/stata9gui/dockfloatpin.html.

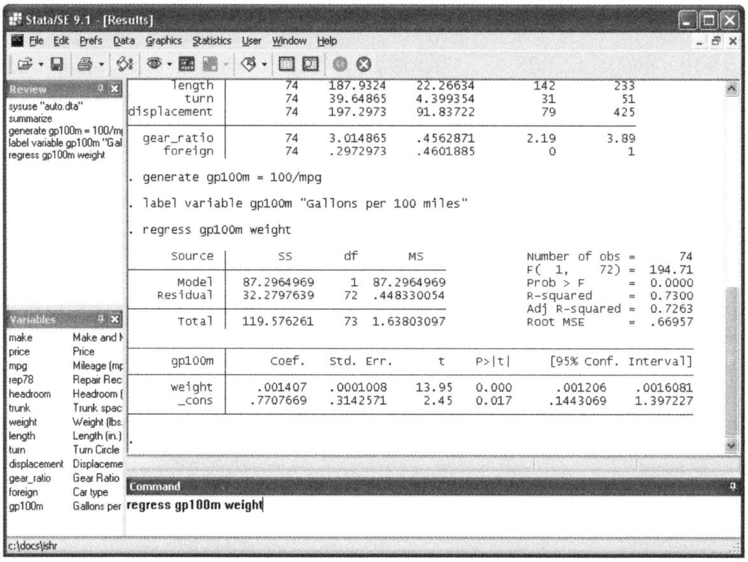

Figure 1.1: Recommended setup of the main windows in Stata

In the lower-left corner, below the Variables window, Stata displays the currently active folder, i.e., the folder where Stata expects files to be located and where files will be saved unless another folder is specified.

Command window

In the Command window, you may enter single commands and execute them by pressing *Enter*.

While reading the rest of this chapter, you might benefit from having opened a dataset. In the Command window, give the command

```
. sysuse auto.dta
```

and see what happens. (`auto` is a dataset included in the installation; such datasets are opened with the `sysuse` command rather than the `use` command.)

Results window

The Results window is the primary display of the output. You may print all or a selected part of the Results window. You can move around using the mouse or the keyboard; to make selections, you must use the mouse.

When the screen is full, it stops to let you read it, displaying `more` at the bottom of the screen. When you press the *Enter* key, the next line is displayed; if you press any other key, the next full screen is displayed. If you dislike the output interruptions by `more`, you can type

```
. set more off
```

or, if you want this setting to be permanent, type

```
. set more off, permanently
```

To activate `more` again, type (do not type the brackets; they mean that `permanently` is optional)

```
. set more on [, permanently]
```

By default, the Results window displays several colors, which can be modified if you wish. It is important that you do not miss error messages, and I chose to let error messages stand out and to underline links:

Prefs ▷ General preferences ▷ Result colors ▷ Color Scheme: Custom 1

Result:	Light yellow
Standard:	Light yellow
Errors:	Strong yellow, bold
Input:	White
Link:	Light blue, underlined
Hilite:	White, bold
Background:	Black

The initial buffer size for the Results window allows for only a few pages of output (32 KB); you may increase it to 200 KB, for example, by typing

```
. set scrollbufsize 200000
```

You must restart Stata for this setting to take effect.

Review window

The Review window displays the most recent commands. Click a command in the Review window to paste it to the Command window, where you may edit and execute it. From the Command window, you may also scroll through past commands using the *PgUp* and *PgDn* keys.

Save past commands to a do-file by right-clicking somewhere in the Review window and selecting **Copy Review Contents to Clipboard**. Next open a Do-file Editor window and paste the Review contents by pressing *Ctrl-V*. See more in section 1.8.

Variables window

The Variables window displays a list of the variables in memory and their labels. Paste a variable name to the Command window by clicking it.

I rarely use variable names of more than 12 characters. To see more of the variable labels in the Variables window, I permanently reduced the space for variable names (default 32 characters) by typing

```
. set varlabelpos 15
```

Some settings in Stata are automatically permanent, and you do not need to specify the `permanently` option. This is one of them.

Viewer window

The main use of the Viewer window (figure 1.2) is viewing help files (see section 2.2). It may also be used to display and print output; see section 1.7. Read more in [GS] **5 Using the Viewer**.

Open the Viewer window by clicking the **Viewer** button, 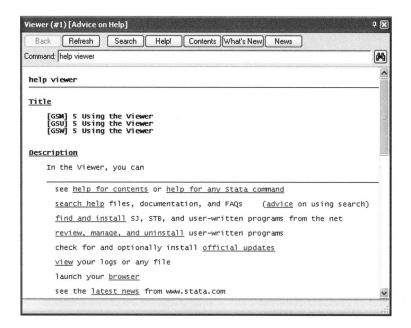. Try the various buttons and see what happens. If the text does not wrap correctly, click the **Refresh** button.

Figure 1.2: The Viewer window

You may have several active Viewer windows simultaneously. You may modify the appearance similarly to the Results window; I chose to underline links as in figure 1.2.

Data Editor/Browser

The Data Editor can be used in two modes. In *browse* mode, you can look at the data without modifying them, while *edit* mode lets you modify and enter data.

The Data Editor looks like a spreadsheet, with variables as columns and observations as rows. String variables are displayed in red and value labels in blue. You may toggle between displaying codes and value labels by right-clicking somewhere in the Data Editor. When the Data Editor is open, you cannot do anything else in Stata, so it does no harm to enlarge the Data Editor to full size and select

> Prefs ▷ Manage preferences ▷ Save preferences

Click the Browse button, ▨ , or type the `browse` command to see data in the Data Browser without the risk of making unintended changes. For example,

`sysuse auto.dta`	Open dataset accompanying Stata
`browse`	All variables, all observations
`browse in 1/5`	All variables, first five observations
`browse make weight length`	Three variables, all observations
`browse make in 23`	The variable `make` in the 23rd observation
`browse mpg if foreign==1`	The variable `mpg`, foreign cars only

To open the Data Editor in edit mode, which allows you to modify data, click the Data Editor button, ▦ . You may now use the Data Editor to enter data; see [GSW] **8 Using the Data Editor**. There are, however, better ways to enter data; see advice in section 6.2. You may also make changes and corrections to the data, but my general recommendation is to make corrections and other permanent modifications to data with a do-file; see section 18.6.

When the Data Editor is open, you cannot do anything else in Stata; close it again to proceed.

Do-file Editor

The Do-file Editor is a standard text editor used for writing text files (typically do-files and ado-files); open it by clicking the Do-file Editor button, ◇ ▾ . The Do-file Editor has the special feature that you may execute all or a selection of the commands by clicking the Do button, ▤↓ , or pressing *Ctrl-D*. The Run button, ▯↓ , is rarely used. Read more in [GSW] **14 Using the Do-file Editor**.

You may check for balanced parentheses. Put the cursor inside a pair of parentheses and press *Ctrl-B*. Try it; it is easier to do than to explain.

Right-click somewhere in a Do-file Editor window to set your preferences, e.g., the font.

You may have several active Do-file Editor windows simultaneously.

1.5   Issuing commands

Using the Command window

In the Command window, you may enter a command and execute it by pressing *Enter*. If the command fails, use *PgUp* to see it again and make modifications. You may also paste a previously used command to the Command window by clicking on the command in the Review window.

Using dialogs to generate commands

The dialogs let you generate complex commands without looking them up in the manuals or the online help. You may need to do some editing if you are not quite satisfied with the result.

There are two ways to activate a dialog. One is to use the menu system to find it; the dialog box for listing observations (the `list` command) is found by selecting

> Data ▷ Describe data ▷ List data

If you know the command name, it is faster to open the dialog box by typing

```
. db list
```

`list` is a simple and often used command, and it is easier to enter it in the Command window, but for graphs and many analyses, the dialogs are a blessing. To understand the opportunities fully, you must, however, have some basic understanding of Stata's command syntax rules; see chapter 4.

Using do-files

A do-file is a series of commands to be executed in sequence. For any major task, this method is preferable to entering single commands because

- You make sure that the commands are executed in the sequence intended.
- If you discover an error, you can easily correct it and rerun the do-file.
- The do-file serves as documentation of what you did.

A do-file is a plain-text (ASCII) file; it might look like the following:

```
                            ─── regress1.do ───
* regress1.do
sysuse auto.dta
generate gp100m = 100/mpg
label variable gp100m "Gallons per 100 miles"
summarize gp100m
regress gp100m weight
rvfplot, yline(0)
```

I always start a do-file with a comment (* `regress1.do`) stating the do-file's name. The next six commands could have been given one by one in the Command window, but together they constitute an analysis, and keeping them together is extremely practical.

Use the Do-file Editor or another text editor to write your do-files.

> Note: the last line in a do-file (and an ado-file) must end with a carriage return, or it will not work. The Do-file Editor automatically takes care of that, but if you use another text editor, you must include a carriage return yourself.

The do command

Find and execute a do-file by selecting

> File ▷ Do...

or by entering the path and filename in the Command window:

```
. do "C:\docs\proj1\regress1.do"
```

If `C:\docs\proj1` is the current folder (look at the Stata screen's lower-left corner), you need to enter only

```
. do regress1.do
```

You can use the `cd` command (see section 6.1) to change the current folder:

```
. cd "C:\docs\proj1"
```

From the Do-file Editor, you may also execute the current do-file or a selected part of it by clicking the Do button, , or pressing *Ctrl-D*. This method is easy but has the disadvantage that the do-file is not identified by name but rather by the name of a temporary file.

The Run button, , corresponds to the `run` command; it executes the commands without displaying any output. You will rarely want to use it.

1.6 Exercises

The purpose of these exercises is to guide you through the customization process and help you become familiar with the user interface. In section 1.9, you will find more exercises concerning methods to handle output.

1-1. If you have not installed Stata, do it now (see section 1.1).

1-2. If you have not updated Stata, do it now (see section 1.1).

1-3. Use Explorer or My Computer to create the folder C:\docs\ishr; you will use it for the exercises. (You may, of course, decide on another location, but in this book's examples, I assume that C:\docs is your personal main folder.) At the web site http://www.stata-press.com/data/ishr.html, you will find instructions on how to download the datasets used in this book. Also, create the folders C:\ado and C:\ado\personal if they do not already exist.

1-4. If you have not already done so, organize Stata's windows as shown in section 1.4. Once you have the windows organized as desired, save your preferences by selecting

Prefs ▷ Manage preferences ▷ Save preferences

1-5. In the Command window, enter

. **sysuse auto.dta**

This command reads a dataset that is installed with Stata. Note that commands must be entered in lowercase as shown; Stata does not understand Sysuse or SYSUSE.

Look at the Variables window; it displays the names of variables in the auto.dta dataset.

1-6. Open the Data Browser by typing the command

. **browse**

and take a look. You might want to modify the window size or the font. If you do, remember to save your preferences by selecting

Prefs ▷ Manage preferences ▷ Save preferences

Now close the Data Browser. Open it again to see the values of make, mpg, and foreign for the first five observations by typing

. **browse make mpg foreign in 1/5**

make (a string variable) is displayed in red, while the value labels for foreign are displayed in blue. Right-click somewhere in the Data Editor window to toggle between value labels and codes for foreign.

You can click a button to open the Data Browser, too, , but you will not be able to select observations and variables.

1-7. In the Command window, enter

. **summarize**

and look at the Results window. summarize displays the number of valid observations and the mean, standard deviation, and minimum and maximum values of all variables.

Use the mouse to highlight the table, and print it. (Click the **Print** button. In the dialog that appears, click the **Selection** radio button.)

1-8. Look at the Review window, which displays the two commands issued so far (and possibly some errors you made). Now click the last command (summarize) to copy it to the Command window. In the Variables window, click mpg to copy it to the Command window, which now displays

> . summarize mpg

Press the *Enter* key, and see what happens.

1-9. Try using the dialog system to obtain the same result. If you know the command name, it is easiest to enter the db (dialog box) command:

> . db summarize

If you are searching for a command but do not know its name, use the menu system; for summarize, select

> Statistics ▷ Summaries, tables & tests ▷ Summary statistics ▷
> Summary statistics

In the dialog that appears, use the drop-down list in the Variables field, and select mpg. Click the OK button. Now you see that the same command you did before is executed.

The dialogs generate commands. For summarize mpg, it obviously is easier to type the command than to create it using the dialog, but for complex commands and graphs, the dialogs are an advantage. In this book, I rarely describe how to use a dialog; instead, I show commands that you can enter by using the Command window, a do-file, or the dialog system.

1-10. Right-click somewhere in the Review window, and select Copy Review Contents to Clipboard. Next paste the text in a Do-file Editor window by typing *Ctrl-V*. If you find any errors, edit the file, and type on the first line clear; your do-file text should look like the following:

```
clear
sysuse auto.dta
summarize
summarize mpg
```

Save the revised do-file as test1.do. Now click the Do-file Editor's Do button, ▤↓ , and see what happens. In the Results window, you will see output like the following:

> . do "C:\Temp\STD00000000.tmp"
>
> . clear
>
> . sysuse auto.dta
> (1978 Automobile Data)

```
. summarize
```

Variable	Obs	Mean	Std. Dev.	Min	Max
make	0				
price	74	6165.257	2949.496	3291	15906
mpg	74	21.2973	5.785503	12	41
...	...				

This process was easy, but the name of the do-file was not displayed. To document your
work, try instead to execute it from the Command window:

```
. do "C:\docs\ishr\test1.do"
```

Instead of specifying the full path for each file, you can specify the file path by using the
cd command (see section 6.1):

```
. cd "C:\docs\ishr"
. do test1.do
```

Rather than remembering the exact path and name of the do-file, it may be easier to find
it by selecting

> File ▷ Do...

1.7   Managing output

This section describes how to manage the output, primarily for printing. If you are a newcomer
to Stata, you might want to skip sections 1.7–1.9 for now and return to them later. But do not
wait too long; the sections include useful tools for handling Stata output.

The output log file

You can have Stata write a copy of the output you see in the Results window to an output log
file; see [GSW] **16 Logs: Printing and saving output** and [U] **15 Printing and preserving
output**. Activate an output log file by typing one of the following commands:

```
. log using logfilename, replace   Overwrite old log file
. log using logfilename, append    Append to existing log file
```

You can suspend logging by typing

```
. log off
```

and resume logging by typing

```
. log on
```

You can also stop logging by typing

```
. log close
```

The output log can be written in two formats: SMCL,[2] which can be displayed by the Viewer only, and plain ASCII text, which can be displayed by a text editor, a word processor, or the Viewer. Select the format by choosing the filename extension:

```
. log using "C:\stata.smcl", replace     SMCL format for display in the Viewer
. log using "C:\stata.log", replace      Text format for display in a text editor
```

You can see the current log status by typing

```
. log
```

The Log button, &♣, lets you open, close, and view the output log file. *Ctrl-L* has the same effect.

If you installed the programs accompanying this book (see the book's web page, http://www.stata-press.com/books/ishr.html), you can discard the current output log and open a new log with the same name by typing

```
. newlog
```

See section 17.5 if you want to know how `newlog` works.

Commands to be executed at program start: profile.do

If you are an inexperienced user, the easiest strategy is to open an output log file at program start. Some experienced users prefer to open a new output log file for each new major task, but my advice is to let Stata open a default output log file when you start the program.

If you have a `profile.do` file (read [GS] **Appendix A.7** for a description) in the *ado-path*, the commands will be executed automatically when you open Stata. Let `profile.do` open an output log file (`stata.log` or `stata.smcl`) and a command log file (`cmdlog.txt`). Write your `profile.do` using Stata's Do-file Editor, and save it in the `C:\ado\personal` folder.[3]

If you want to inspect the output log in the Viewer, taking advantage of the SMCL formatting, create the following `profile.do`:

```
──────────── C:\ado\personal\profile.do ────────────
* C:\ado\personal\profile.do
log using "C:\stata.smcl", replace     // open output log (smcl)
cmdlog using "C:\cmdlog.txt", append   // open command log
```

---

2. SMCL (Stata Markup and Control Language) is much like HTML and is used for formatting help files and for formatting output to be displayed in the Viewer window.

3. [GSW] **Appendix A.7** recommends saving `profile.do` elsewhere. I stick to my recommendation; this folder is safer, as it keeps your `profile.do` stored away from your analysis do-files.

`log` opens Stata's output log file (`stata.smcl`) when the session starts and logs the full output; the `replace` option overwrites output from the previous Stata session. If you want to inspect the output in a text editor, the SMCL formatting is useless, and the second line in `profile.do` should be

```
log using "C:\stata.log", replace      // open output log (text)
```

I prefer the text format because it gives you much more freedom when handling the output.

`cmdlog` opens Stata's command log file (`cmdlog.txt`) to receive the commands issued; the `append` option keeps the command log from previous sessions and lets you examine and reuse past commands. The command log file is described in section 1.8.

Inspecting output in the Viewer window

If you let `profile.do` create the output log file `C:\stata.smcl`, you can open it in the Viewer by typing

```
. view "C:\stata.smcl"
```

You can also click the Log button, ✎, or press *Ctrl-L* to inspect the output log.

In the Viewer, you can select text (using the mouse, not the keyboard) and print it. If the Viewer does not display the most recent output, click the **Refresh** button. You cannot edit the contents of the Viewer.

Inspecting output in a text editor

Any text editor can be used to examine output. Compared with using the Viewer, the advantage of using a text editor is that you can remove errors and mistakes before printing and add comments to the output, so you have more freedom when working with the output. If you want to use a text editor to inspect output, let `profile.do` create `C:\stata.log` (text format); see above.

You can find a thorough assessment of several text editors in a FAQ by Cox (2005) by typing

```
. findit text editors
```

My favorite text editor is NoteTab Light, which you can download for free. You can find a short description and a link to its web site at the author's web site; see *Other supplementary materials provided by the author* at http://www.stata-press.com/books/ishr.html. A major advantage of this editor is that you have access to several files simultaneously; each file has its own tab, hence the name. Section 17.5 shows the `nlog` command as an example of how you can use a third-party text editor—in this case, NoteTab Light—to inspect output. Find `nlog.ado` at this book's web site (http://www.stata-press.com/books/ishr.html).

Copying output to a word-processor document

From the Results window, the Viewer window, or a text editor, you may copy and paste a highlighted part of the output to a word-processor document. To align the text correctly, you must select a monospaced font in the word processor, e.g., Lucida Console 9 pt.

For many tables, you can obtain a more sophisticated result. You can copy results directly to a word-processor document as an HTML table, or you can use Microsoft Excel (or another spreadsheet program) as an intermediary. This method works best if the output is arranged in nice columns.

To copy results as an HTML table, do the following:

1. Highlight the table in the Results window. Right-click the mouse and select Copy Table as HTML.

2. Paste the table into your word-processor document. Once it is there, you should be able to right-click on it to format the cells.

To copy results using a spreadsheet program, do the following:

1. Highlight the table in the Results window. Right-click the mouse and select Copy Table.

2. Open Excel, and paste the table into it (*Ctrl-V*). Format the table if needed, e.g., by adjusting the number of decimals (you will need to use Excel's formatting tools).

3. Copy and paste the table from Excel to your word-processor document.

Decimal periods and commas

To copy output correctly, you must set both Windows and Stata to display decimals as periods or display decimals as commas. To display commas in Stata, type `set dp comma`. To return to the default decimal periods, type `set dp period`. This setting affects only how values are displayed.

Stata commands always use decimal periods, and Stata cannot read or write ASCII data with decimal commas, regardless of the `dp` setting and the Windows settings (see section 6.3), so you should use decimal periods consistently. This is the default in Stata; in Windows, you can change the setting by selecting

[Start] ▷ Settings ▷ Control Panel ▷ Regional and Language Options

Here you can choose a country that uses decimal periods.

If you are creating a graph and want axis labels with decimal commas, `set dp comma`.

1.8   Reusing commands

As shown in section 1.4, the Review window displays the most recent commands issued. Click a command to paste it to the Command window. Copy all the commands to the Windows clipboard by right-clicking somewhere in the Review window and selecting Copy Review Contents to Clipboard.

Next, open a Do-file Editor window and paste the text with *Ctrl-V*. The do-file will probably need some editing.

You can have Stata copy all future commands within the current session to a command log file by typing

> . **cmdlog using** *cmdlogfilename* [**, replace** | **append**]

The command log is always plain text. If you, as we suggested in section 1.7, had `profile.do` generate a command log file (`C:\cmdlog.txt`), you can inspect it in the Do-file Editor. You can also copy and paste a group of commands to a new window, edit them, and save a revised do-file. Since we set the command log file to be cumulative (the `append` option), you can even access commands from previous sessions. Using a log this way is a good alternative to copying the Review window contents to the Do-file Editor. The `ecmd` command (see section 17.5) opens the command log in the Do-file Editor.

An extended `profile.do`, shown in section 17.5, adds a time stamp to the cumulative command log when a new session starts to help you find past commands.

1.9 More exercises

The following exercises relate to sections 1.7 and 1.8 and are designed to give you some experience with methods of handling the output.

1-11. If you have not done so already, create a `profile.do` as described in section 1.7. You must restart Stata to use the file.

1-12. Do some of the exercises with the `auto` dataset in section 1.6 to create some output to work with. Next, press *Ctrl-L*, and select View snapshot of log file. The output (`stata.log` or `stata.smcl`) from the entire session is now displayed in a Viewer window. Here you can use the mouse to select what you want to print, but you cannot edit anything. You can also copy parts of the output to your word processor (select a fixed-width font in the word processor to make the tables align correctly).

If you have installed a text editor, such as NoteTab Light, you may use it for output. Here you can edit it, remove junk, add comments, etc., and send a selection to the printer. The `nlog` command, available at this book's web site, lets you open the output log in NoteTab Light.

1-13. In a Do-file Editor window, open `C:\cmdlog.txt` (the command log). This file displays the commands issued, and it can be used the same way you used the Review window in exercises 1–10 to generate a do-file of past commands. Select a group of commands, and copy and paste them to a new Do-file Editor window. Here you can edit the commands and save a workable do-file: `test2.do` in `C:\docs\ishr`. Run this do-file (File ▷ Do...).

2 Getting help—and more

2.1 The manuals

For beginners, this book and the *Getting Started* manual might suffice, but this book does not replace the manuals; they have much more detail and documentation than could be written in this book. [GSW], [U], [D], etc., refer to the official manuals:

[GS]   *Getting Started* gives an overview of Stata's main features. [GSW] is for the Windows version; there are similar introductions to the Unix and Macintosh versions as well.

[U]   *User's Guide* gives a systematic description of Stata.

[D]   *Data Management Reference Manual* includes commands for reading and saving files, making calculations, and modifying the data structure.

[R]   *Base Reference Manual* (three volumes) includes all general commands, except those in [D].

[ST]   *Survival Analysis and Epidemiological Tables Reference Manual* includes descriptive procedures, survival regression models, and procedures for the analysis of epidemiological tables.

[G]   *Graphics Reference Manual* includes information about Stata's graphics.

[I]   *Quick Reference and Index Manual* includes brief descriptions of Stata procedures and an index.

There are more manuals than these; see more on manuals and other useful books in appendix A.

2.2 Online help

Keeping your Stata updated will update your online help, too. To read more about the online help, see [GSW] **6 Help** and [U] **4 Stata's online help and search facilities**; most of it works as you would expect. See also [R] **net** and [R] **search**.

help

The `help` command displays information in the Viewer window; you can also type `help` at the Viewer command line.

If you know a command name (e.g., `tabstat`), you can display a help file (`tabstat.hlp`) by typing `help` *command_name*, for example,

    `. help tabstat`

You can get the same result by clicking

      Help ▷ Stata Command...

and typing `tabstat`.

The help file is displayed in the Viewer window, and from here you may print it. You may also use the links included; try it. For more information on the contents and interpretation of syntax diagrams and online help, see section 4.2.

You can also find help for functions, for example, the `exp()` (exponential) function:

    `. help exp()`

`help` displays information stored on your own computer, but you can also find help on the Internet too, as you will see.

Using the menus and dialogs

If you are searching for a command, a good strategy is to use the menus and dialogs. Suppose that you want to find out about Stata's facilities concerning nonparametric statistics:

      Statistics ▷ Summaries, tables, & tests ▷ Nonparametric tests of hypotheses

This sequence displays a menu with (currently) 11 tests. If you select a test, for example, Kruskal–Wallis rank test, Stata opens a dialog. Click the ? button in the dialog's lower-left corner to see the online help for the `kwallis` command.

search

You can find information about a command even if you do not know the command name.

For example, you can get information about nonparametric tests by typing

    `. search nonparametric`

You can get the same result by clicking

      Help ▷ Search...

and typing `nonparametric`.

This search lists refers to several official Stata entries:

- Help files on your computer for several Stata commands

- FAQs (frequently asked questions; see section 2.3)

- Papers and programs published in the SJ (*Stata Journal*) and its predecessor, the STB (*Stata Technical Bulletin*)

The Help ▷ Search... dialog also lets you search outside the official Stata; this dialog corresponds to the commands

```
. search nonparametric, net     Searches official and unofficial web sites
. search nonparametric, all     Searches your computer and all web sites
```

Unofficial web sites include several commands (ado-files) and papers generated by creative users. The largest such site is SSC (Statistical Software Components) at Boston College. Read more in [R] **ssc** or

```
. help ssc
```

The number of unofficial ado-files available may seem overwhelming, but I often find what I am looking for. One problem with unofficial programs is that there is no formal quality control. Errors do occur, even in the official programs, but Stata has formal procedures to ensure corrections once an error has been detected. To check for updates to unofficial commands you have installed on your computer, type

```
. adoupdate
```

findit

An easy alternative to search ..., all is the findit command:

```
. findit nonparametric
```

Say that you are looking for a command that estimates sensitivity, specificity, and predictive values for a binary diagnostic test. You will want to include keywords that are likely to identify all relevant commands (a sensitivity issue) without pointing to too many irrelevant commands (the specificity problem). I chose

```
. findit sensitivity specificity
```

and found, among other things,

```
SJ-4-4  sbe36_2 . . . . . . . . . . . . . . . . . . Software update for diagt
        (help diagt if installed) . . . . . . . . . P. T. Seed and A. Tobias
        Q4/04   SJ 4(4):490
        new options added to diagt
```

Currently no official Stata command does what we want, but the unofficial command `diagt` seems to. Information on this procedure was published in the *Stata Journal*, volume 4, number 4. Click the link `sbe36_2` to obtain

```
package sbe36_2 from http://www.stata-journal.com/software/sj4-4
```

```
TITLE
      SJ4-4 sbe36_2.  Summary statistics for diagnostic tests

DESCRIPTION/AUTHOR(S)
      Summary statistics for diagnostic tests
      by Paul T. Seed, King's College London, UK
         Aurelio Tobias, Universidad Carlos III de Madrid, Spain
      Support:  paul.seed@kcl.ac.uk, atobias@wanadoo.es
      After installation, type help diagt and diagti

INSTALLATION FILES                          (click here to install)
      sbe36_2/diagt.ado
      sbe36_2/diagt.hlp
      sbe36_2/diagti.ado
      sbe36_2/diagti.hlp
```

```
(click here to return to the previous screen)
```

Now click the link `click here to install`; next read the help file. The use of the `diagt` command is illustrated in section 15.3. Unofficial programs are automatically installed in `C:\ado\plus`.

2.3   Other resources

For an overview of available resources, see [U] **3 Resources for learning and using Stata**.

Stata NetCourses

Stata offers NetCourses to newcomers and advanced users. Read more about NetCourses at http://www.stata.com/netcourse.

FAQs

Stata's web site includes a lot of advice on various topics, including several FAQs (frequently asked questions; http://www.stata.com/support/faqs/). You may look for information using the structured list of contents, or you may perform a keyword search.

Say that you are uncertain about Stata's handling of missing values and want to see if there is an FAQ on the subject. Open http://www.stata.com/support/faqs/, and enter `missing values` in the search field. Among the articles listed you may find this one promising: *Why is x > 1000 true when x contains missing value?* You would be led to the same FAQ (among many other items) if you typed

```
. findit missing values
```

Statalist

Statalist is a users' forum for exchange of questions, answers, advice, and ideas; see

```
. help statalist
```

Stata technical support

You can email Stata and ask for help. You should, however, try to help yourself first by looking up the relevant information in the online help and the manuals. You can find good advice before emailing by typing

```
. search technical support
```

If you believe you have found an error, by all means write to technical support. You may be right, but even if you are not, you will get a swift and informative answer. If possible, include a small dataset and a do-file demonstrating the problem.

Asking a more experienced user

The same considerations as above apply. Assuming that the more experienced user really wants to help you, consider what information the user will need. If you do not understand why something does not work, include output with commands and error messages.

2.4   Errors and error messages

Stata's short error messages include a code, e.g., $r(131)$. The code is a link, which you can click to get more information about the error. Designing useful error messages, however, is complicated, and Stata cannot always guess your intent, so you may not always find the error message to be helpful. The following sections discuss frequent errors and the corresponding error messages.

Stata is case sensitive

Remember that Stata is case sensitive; this applies both to Stata commands and variables:

```
. List
unrecognized command:  List
r(199);
```

Stata told you that it did not recognize the List command. Click the $r(199)$ link to get more details:

```
[P]    error . . . . . . . . . . . . . . . . . . . . . . . . . . Return code 199
       unrecognized command;
       Stata failed to recognize the command, program, or ado-file name,
       probably because of a typographical or abbreviation error.
```

The details are not informative, but you probably wanted to use the `list` command, which is spelled `list`, not `List`.

The == equal sign in relational expressions

Remember the difference between the assignment equal sign (=) and the relational equal sign (==); see section 4.4:

```
. summarize if foreign = 1
invalid syntax
r(198);
```

To get more information, click the `r(198)` link; it is not informative, either. The actual error was that you were using the single equal sign in a relational expression, but it should have been

```
. summarize if foreign == 1
```

Commas and options

Misplacing the comma preceding options is a frequent beginner's error (although experienced users do it, too):

```
. summarize, if foreign==1
option if not allowed
r(198);
```

Stata interprets everything after a comma as an option. `summarize` has no `if` option. You probably wanted to use the `if` qualifier, which must be placed before any comma (see sections 4.4 and 4.5), and the command should have been

```
. summarize if foreign==1
```

Forgetting the comma is common, too:

```
. ttest price by(foreign)
time-series operators not allowed
r(101);
```

This error message was not helpful; you really did not do anything that should make Stata think of time-series analysis. However, `by()` is an option of `ttest`, so it should be preceded by a comma, and the command should have been

```
. ttest price, by(foreign)
```

Space between option names and arguments

There is no space between an option name and a subsequent parenthesis. Stata often forgives a space, but not always; the error message may be confusing:

```
. scatter mpg weight, xtitle ("Weight")
"Weight invalid name
invalid syntax
r(198);
. scatter mpg weight, xtitle (Weight)
option xtitle() not allowed
invalid syntax
r(198);
```

In both cases, there was an inappropriate space between `xtitle` and the parenthesis containing the argument. Both commands below are correct:

```
. scatter mpg weight, xtitle("Weight")
. scatter mpg weight, xtitle(Weight)
```

Especially in complex graph commands, such errors may be difficult to identify.

3 Stata file types and names

Stata works with several types of files; the most important are shown below. The filename extension shows the file type, both to the user and to the operating system:

```
. use alpha.dta    Opens Stata dataset
. do alpha.do      Executes Stata do-file
```

Often Stata allows you to omit the filename extension:

```
. use alpha        Opens Stata dataset
. do alpha         Executes Stata do-file
```

However, including the filename extension makes the command more transparent, and I will do that throughout this book. This advice is consistent with my advice to let Windows display filename extensions; see appendix B.

Quotes should be used if a filename includes spaces.

.dta files: Stata data

The extension for a Stata dataset is `.dta`. Stata datasets can be interpreted only by Stata and by programs specifically designed to read Stata datasets, such as Stat/Transfer.

.do-files: command files

A do-file with the extension `.do` is a group of commands to be executed in sequence. Do-files are in plain-text (ASCII) format and can be edited and displayed by any text editor, such as Stata's Do-file Editor.

You can issue single commands in the Command window, but if you are doing anything substantial, you should use a do-file; see section 1.5.

.ado-files: programs

An ado-file with the extension `.ado` is a program. Ado-files are in plain-text format. For more information, see section 17.3.

.hlp files: Stata help

Stata's online documentation is stored in .hlp files, written in SMCL format, which is somewhat like HTML. SMCL-formatted files can be displayed in the Viewer window. (Do not confuse Stata's help files with Windows' .hlp files; if you double-click a Stata .hlp file in Windows Explorer or My Computer, Windows will give you an error message.)

If you look in the Stata folders, you will also see .ihlp files, which contain help that can be reused in several help files.

.gph files: graphs

Stata graphs can be saved as .gph files; see section 11.9.

.txt files: plain ASCII format

A plain-text file simply includes lines of text (the text may also be numbers). The Stata manuals give such files the extension .raw, whereas most other Windows applications, by default, use the extension .txt. In this book, I will use the extension .txt.

.scheme: settings for graphs

To control the appearance of graphs, use the extension .scheme; see section 11.4.

There are more file types than this. For an overview, see [U] **11.6 File-naming conventions**.

4 Command syntax

4.1 General syntax rules

Stata's command syntax rules are described in detail in [U] **11 Language syntax**.

Stata is case sensitive, and almost all Stata commands are lowercase. `list` is a valid command, but `List` is not. Variable names may include lowercase and uppercase letters, but `sex` and `Sex` are two different variable names. Throughout this book, I use lowercase variable names.

Variable names can have 1–32 characters, but Stata often abbreviates long variable names in output, so I recommend using 10 characters at most. The letters a–z, the numbers 0–9, and _ (underscore) are valid characters. Non-English characters like ü, ø, è, and ž are not accepted, or at least not safe. Names must start with a letter (or an underscore, but this is strongly discouraged because many Stata-generated temporary variables start with an underscore). The following are valid variable names:

```
a q17 q_17 pregnant sex
```

4.2 Syntax diagrams

A syntax diagram is a formal description of the elements in a Stata command. The notation used is described in [R] **intro** (in the beginning of the first volume of the *Base Reference* manual).

The general syntax of typical Stata commands can be written like this:

$$\big[\,prefix\!:\,\big]\ command\ \big[\,varlist\,\big]\ \big[\,if\,\big]\ \big[\,in\,\big]\ \big[\,weight\,\big]\ \big[\,,\ options\,\big]$$

(*Continued on next page*)

For example, the syntax for summarize is

$$\underline{su}mmarize\ \big[\,varlist\,\big]\ \big[\,if\,\big]\ \big[\,in\,\big]\ \big[\,weight\,\big]\ \big[\,,\ options\,\big]$$

options	description
Main	
detail	display additional statistics
meanonly	suppress the display; calculate only the mean; (programmer's option)
format	use variable's display format
separator(#)	draw separator line after every # variables; default is separator(5)

varlist may contain time-series operators; see [U] **11.4.3 Time-series varlist**.

by may be used with summarize; see [D] **by**.

aweights, fweights, and iweights are allowed. However, iweights may not be used
   with the detail option; see [U] **11.1.6 weight**.

Thin square brackets, [ ], mean that the item is optional, so the only mandatory part of the
summarize syntax is the command name itself. Square brackets may also be part of the syntax,
in which case they are shown in ordinary typewriter font, as in

```
tab2 case ctrl [fweight=pop]
```

Curly brackets, { }, mean that you must specify one of the options, but not both options, as
in

$$numlabel\ \big[\,lblname\text{-}list\,\big],\ \big\{\,\underline{a}dd\,|\,\underline{re}move\,\big\}$$

Here you must specify either add or remove. Command and option names may be abbreviated; underlining shows the minimum abbreviation. I use few abbreviations because although
they make commands faster to write, they are difficult to read.

Here are some example `summarize` commands:

prefix	command	varlist	qualifiers/weights	options	comments
	summarize	_all			_all: all variables
	summarize				All variables
	sum				Abbreviated
	summarize	sex age			Two variables
	summarize	sex-weight			Variable range
	summarize	pro*			All variables starting with pro
	summarize	*ro*			All variables including ro
	summarize	??ro?			5-letter variables, ro 3rd and 4th characters
	summarize	age	if sex==1		Males only
	summarize	bmi	in 1/10		First 10 observations
	summarize	bmi	[fweight=n]		Weighted observations
	sort	sex			Separate table for each
by sex:	summarize	bmi			sex. Data must be sorted first.
	summarize	bmi		, detail	Option: detail

Below is the online help for `summarize`, which is displayed in the Viewer window by typing

    `. help summarize`

(*Continued on next page*)

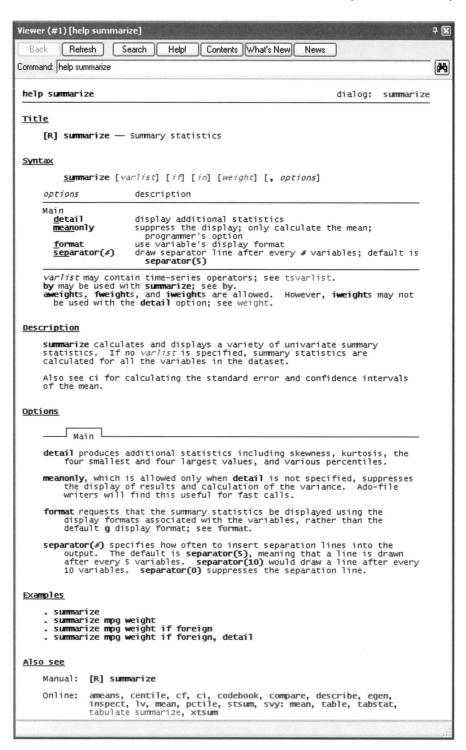

The help description includes several links to related commands and other information. Compared with the information in the *Base Reference manual*, the online help is brief. The manuals typically include more elaborate examples, a description of statistical methods, and references.

4.3 Lists of variables and numbers

Variable lists

A variable list (*varlist*) defines one or more variables to be processed; see [U] **11.1.1 varlist**. Examples:

(nothing)	Sometimes means the same as _all
_all	All variables in the dataset
sex age pregnant	Three variables
pregnant sex-weight	pregnant and the consecutive variables from sex to weight
pro*	All variables starting with pro
ro	All variables including ro
??ro?	5-letter variables with ro as third and fourth character

When generating new variables, you may refer to the 17 variables q1, q2, ..., q17 as q1-q17. When referring to the existing variables q1-q17, you will get q1, q17, and the variables that come between them in the dataset, but they are not necessarily the 15 variables q2, q3, ..., q16. summarize and describe are useful commands to see the ordering of variables in the dataset.

In commands that have a dependent variable, it is the first in the variable list:

. oneway bmi sex	bmi is the dependent variable
. regress bmi sex age	bmi is the dependent variable
. scatter weight height	Scatterplot, weight is the y-axis
. tab2 expos case	The first variable defines the rows

Numeric lists

A numeric list (*numlist*) is a list of numbers with some shorthand possibilities (see [U] **11.1.8 numlist**):

1(3)11	means	1 4 7 10
1(1)4 4.5(0.5)6	means	1 2 3 4 4.5 5 5.5 6
4 3 2 7(-1)1	means	4 3 2 7 6 5 4 3 2 1
1/5	means	1 2 3 4 5
4/2 7/1	means	4 3 2 7 6 5 4 3 2 1

Numeric lists have many uses, for example,

- Display person-time and incidence rates every 0.5 years, up to 5 years:

      . stptime, at(0(0.5)5) by(drug)

- Graph with y-axis labels at 0 10 20 30 40:

      . scatter mpg weight, ylabel(0(10)40)

- Age groups 0–4, 5–14, 15–24, …, 75–84, 85+:

      . egen agegrp = cut(age), at(0 5(10)85 200)

Numeric ranges

Numeric lists should not be confused with numeric ranges. The following are ranges:

      . list in 1/10
      . recode age (0/24=1)(25/44=2)(45/max=3), generate(agegr)

4.4   Qualifiers

Qualifiers are common to many commands, while most options are specific to one or a few commands.

The if qualifier

The if qualifier is used in logical expressions to select the observations to which a command applies; see [U] **11.1.3 if exp**. Below are a few examples:

. summarize age if sex == 1	Males only
. summarize age if sex != 1	Males excluded
. list id age if age <= 25	Young only
. replace npreg=. if sex==1	Males: npreg missing
. list sex age weight if sex == 1 & age <= 25	Young males only
. keep if sex == 1 | age <= 25	Males or young
. keep if !(sex == 1 | age <= 25)	All others

Two types of operators are used in logical expressions; see [U] **13.2 Operators**:

Relational operators		Logical operators	
>	Greater than	!	Not
<	Less than	~	Not
>=	Greater than or equal	&	And
<=	Less than or equal	|	Or
==	Equal		
!=	Not equal		
~=	Not equal		

The double equal sign "==" in relational expressions has a meaning different from that of the assignment equal sign as in

```
. generate bmi = weight/(height^2)
```

Logical expressions are evaluated to true or false; a value of 0 means false, and any other value, including missing values, means true. Technically, missing values are large positive numbers and are evaluated as such in logical expressions; see [U] **12.2.1 Missing values**. This behavior leads to this warning:

WARNING! Missing values in logical expressions.

The following command initially surprised me by listing all whose ages were greater than 65 and those with missing age:

```
. list id age if age > 65
```

Technically, a missing value is larger than any valid number, which means that the expression age > 65 is true if age is missing. To exclude the missing values, type

```
. list id age if age > 65 & age < .
```

or

```
. list id age if age>65 & !missing(age)
```

To list the missing values only, including user-defined missing values, type

```
. list id age if age >=.
```

or

```
. list id age if missing(age)
```

See [U] **12.2.1 Missing values** for more information.

In the `auto.dta` dataset, the variable `foreign` takes the values 0 and 1. You may see a construct like

```
. keep if foreign
```

`foreign` can be evaluated as a logical expression, being false if `foreign` is 0 and true otherwise. I find this method a bit dangerous because any observations with `foreign` missing would be included, too, and that might not be what you intended.

With complex logical expressions, use parentheses to control the order of evaluation:

```
. anycommand if ((sex==1 & weight>90) | (sex==2 & weight>80))
> & weight<.
```

Omitting the parentheses might give a different selection, but that outcome may be difficult to predict. Use parentheses to make the syntax transparent to yourself; then it will work correctly. Another way to handle complex selections is to generate a help variable (`heavy`):

`. generate heavy=0`	Initialize help variable
`. replace heavy=1 if sex==1 & weight>90`	Include males > 90 kg
`. replace heavy=1 if sex==2 & weight>80`	Include females > 80 kg
`. replace heavy=. if weight >=.`	Don't include if `weight` is missing
`. anycommand if heavy==1`	These are the heavy ones

The in qualifier

The `in` qualifier is used to select the observations to which a command applies; see [U] **11.1.4 in range**. It is especially useful for listing or displaying a subset of observations. Below are three examples:

`. list sex age weight in 23`	23rd observation
`. list in 1/10`	All variables; observations 1–10
`. browse sex-weight in -5/-1`	See last 5 observations in the Data Browser

The last observation is identified by `-1`, and `-5/-1` means the last 5 observations.

4.5   Weights

Weighting observations

Weights may be used to "multiply" observations when the input is tabular; see [U] **11.1.6 weight**. Suppose that you see the following table in a paper and want to analyze it further.

	Cases	Controls
Exposed	21	30
Unexposed	23	100
Total	44	130

The `input` command (see section 6.2) lets you enter the tabular data directly:

```
. input expos case pop
1 1 21
1 0 30
0 1 23
0 0 100
end
```

Now you can analyze the data by weighting with pop:

```
. tab2 expos case [fweight=pop], chi2
. cc expos case [fweight=pop]
```

The square brackets around the weight expression are part of the syntax; here they do not indicate options.

`fweight` indicates frequency weighting. For information about other types of weighting, see [U] **20.16 Weighted estimation**.

Instead of weighting the analysis, you could `expand` the dataset; see section 9.5.

4.6 Options

Options are specific to a command, and you must look in the manuals or the online help to see the options that are available; see [U] **11.1.7 options**. Options come last in the command; they are preceded by a comma. Usually, there is only one comma per command, but complex graph commands may include more; see chapter 11.

The `nolabel` option is common to many commands. If value labels have been assigned to a variable, Stata usually displays the value label rather than the code in tables and listings. The `nolabel` option lets you see the code but not the label:

```
. sysuse auto, clear
(1978 Automobile Data)

. tab1 foreign

-> tabulation of foreign

   Car type |      Freq.     Percent        Cum.
------------+-----------------------------------
   Domestic |         52       70.27       70.27
    Foreign |         22       29.73      100.00
------------+-----------------------------------
      Total |         74      100.00
```

```
. tab1 foreign, nolabel

-> tabulation of foreign
    Car type |      Freq.     Percent        Cum.
-------------+-----------------------------------
           0 |         52       70.27       70.27
           1 |         22       29.73      100.00
-------------+-----------------------------------
       Total |         74      100.00
```

The same applies to browsing (looking at the Data window):

> `. browse displacement-foreign in 1/2`   Display any labels
> `. browse displacement-foreign in 1/2, nolabel`   Display codes

In the Data window, you may toggle between codes and value labels (blue text) by right-clicking somewhere in the Data window.

The `missing` option is common to many commands. It means that missing codes are included in tabulations, etc., like any other category.

The `level()` option is common to many commands. It is used to specify confidence levels other than the default 95%. You could specify 90% confidence intervals by typing

> `. regress mpg weight, level(90)`

4.7 Prefixes

Only the by *varlist:* prefix is shown here, but there are others, e.g., `xi:` (see section 13.1).

The by varlist: prefix

See [U] **11.5 by varlist: construct**. The by *varlist:* prefix makes a command perform calculations or display results for strata of the data. Data must be sorted by the stratification variables. The following commands lead to two `summarize` tables, one for each sex:

> `. sort sex`
> `. by sex: summarize age height weight`

You can produce the same results with a single command:

> `. by sex, sort: summarize age height weight`

4.8 Other syntax elements

Text strings, quotes

Stata requires double quotes around text strings that contain embedded blank spaces or commas:

```
. label define sex  1 male  2 female  9 "sex unknown"
```

You need not use quotes around filenames and file paths, such as

```
. save alpha1.dta
```

unless they include a blank space:

```
. save "alpha 1.dta"
```

Comments

See [U] **16.1.2 Comments and blank lines in do-files**. The following are interpreted as comments, so you can include short explanations in do-files and ado-files:

- Lines beginning with *
- Text surrounded by /* and */
- Text following //

Comments make your do-files more readable; Stata does not care what you write:

```
* C:\ado\personal\profile.do executes when opening Stata
summarize bmi, detail          // Body mass index
```

The above applies to do-files and ado-files. In the Command window, you may enter a comment with *, but not with // or /*...*/.

Long lines in do-files and ado-files

See [U] **16.1.3 Long lines in do-files**. In do-files and ado-files, a command, by default, ends when the line ends (carriage return), and no special delimiter terminates commands. However, command lines in do-files and ado-files should be no longer than 80 characters for readability on most screens. This problem is solved by typing /// to indicate that the following line is a continuation.

```
infix str10 cprstr 1-10 bday 1-2 bmon 3-4 byear 5-6    ///
      control 7-10 using datefile.txt
```

Another option is to define ; (the semicolon) as the future command delimiter:

```
#delimit ;                 // Semicolon delimits future commands

infix str10 cprstr 1-10 bday 1-2 bmon 3-4 byear 5-6
      control 7-10 using "datefile.txt";
tab1 byear;

#delimit cr                // Back to normal: Carriage return delimiter
```

Text enclosed by /* and */ is also interpreted as a comment; it can then be used to "comment out" a carriage return:

```
infix str10 cprstr 1-10 bday 1-2 bmon 3-4 byear 5-6    /*
    */ control 7-10 using "datefile.txt"
```

> **NOTE:** The above does not apply to commands entered in the Command window; here you just continue writing the command until you are finished and hit *Enter.* In the Command window, the // comment characters and the /// continuation characters are not allowed, but you may use * to insert a comment.

In output, a long command entered in the Command window will be displayed like this:

```
. infix str10 cprstr 1-10 bday 1-2 bmon 3-4 byear 5-6 control 7-10
> using "datefile.txt"
```

Abbreviating command, option, and variable names

See [U] **11.2 Abbreviation rules**. In commands, you may abbreviate variable names to the minimum number of characters that unambiguously identify the variable. As shown in section 4.2, you may also abbreviate command and option names. This means that the command

```
. summarize age if sex==1, detail
```

can be abbreviated to

```
. su a if s==1, d
```

unless there are other variables in the dataset starting with a or s.

I rarely use abbreviations; it is more important that the command be easy to read than easy to write, and with abbreviations, the risk of mistakes is rather high. You may develop your private habits, but try to make the syntax readable when communicating with others (please!). If you look at or participate in the exchanges at Statalist (see section 2.3), you might meet syntax like

```
. qui su
```

This might make no sense whatsoever to you, but fortunately the help system understands the abbreviations, so typing

```
. help qui
```

tells you that the command is quietly. From here it is easy; the full command is

```
. quietly summarize
```

5 Variables

A Stata dataset is rectangular; here is an example with five observations and four variables:

	Variables			
	obsno	age	height	weight
	1	27	178	74
	2	54	166	67
Observations	3	63	173	85
	4	36	182	81
	5	57	165	90

This corresponds to what you see in Stata's Data window when you issue a `browse` command.

5.1 Types of variables

Stata has two main types of variables: numeric and string. String variables are described in section 5.6. Read more about variable types in [U] **12 Data** and [D] **data types**.

Date variables are a special variety of numeric variables; they are described in section 5.5. A special variety of date variables is time-series dates; they are not described in this book.

For most purposes, numeric variables are more useful than string variables, and some analyses do not work with string variables. Sections 5.2–5.4 deal with numeric variables only. You might decide to postpone reading sections 5.5 and 5.6 until you feel the need.

5.2 Numeric formats

See [U] **12.5.1 Numeric formats** and [D] **format**. Format means display format; a format specification does not affect the values in the dataset, but only the way they are displayed in the output. You can see the formats applied to variables in a dataset by typing

. `describe` [*varlist*]

Format	Formula	Example	$\sqrt{2}$	1,000	10,000,000
General	%*w.d*g	%9.0g	1.414214	1000	1.00e+07
Fixed	%*w.d*f	%9.0f	1	1000	10000000
		%9.2f	1.41	1000.00	1.00e+07
		%09.2f	000001.41	001000.00	1.00e+07
Exponential	%*w.d*e	%10.3e	1.414e+00	1.000e+03	1.000e+07

w: The total width, including period and decimals

d: Number of decimals

The default is the g (general) format, displaying values with reasonable precision. Usually, you need not bother with numeric formats, but you may specify a fixed (f) format, e.g.,

```
. format usd eur %10.2f
. format jpy %10.0fc
. list in 1/3, clean
         usd       eur        jpy
  1.   1645.82   1362.40    192,308
  2.  22628.54  18731.74  2,644,058
  3.  12693.05  10507.22  1,483,135
```

For jpy, the c in the format specification displays commas as thousands delimiters.

set dp comma displays decimal commas, but you must still use decimal periods in commands. Displaying decimal commas is probably most relevant for graphs, but here is how it works; it also changes the display of thousands delimiters:

```
. set dp comma
. list in 1/3, clean
         usd       eur        jpy
  1.   1645,82   1362,40    192.308
  2.  22628,54  18731,74  2.644.058
  3.  12693,05  10507,22  1.483.135
```

You may also specify a format as, e.g., %9,0g to display decimal commas, but it does not always work as expected. Remember that no matter how you specify formats, in commands Stata understands only decimal periods.

The general rule is that format affects the display of single values, as in list, whereas output from analyses is displayed regardless of the format. There are, however, exceptions, and a fixed (f) format does influence the output from tabulate with the summarize() option, oneway with the tabulate option, and ci. In some other commands, such as tabstat (section 10.4), a format() option lets you determine the output format.

5.3 Missing values

Missing values are omitted from calculations and analyses. There are two types of missing values:

- *System missing values* are shown as a . (period). Such a value is created in input when a numeric field is empty; by invalid calculations, e.g., division by 0; and by calculations involving a missing value.
- *User-defined missing values* are .a, .b, .c, ..., .z. It is a good idea to use a general principle consistently, e.g.,

.	Question not asked (complications to an operation not performed)
.a	Question asked, no response
.b	Response: Do not know

See [U] **12.2.1 Missing values** and [D] **missing values**. Coding missing information as missing is important for continuous variables. Ask yourself, Would it make any sense to calculate the mean for this variable? If not, as is the case for categorical variables, consider how you want to use information about nonresponses and do-not-know responses in your analyses. A "Do not know" answer is often as interesting as a "Yes", and in such cases do-not-know responses should not be coded as missing.

If you enter data in Stata's Data Editor, you may also enter these missing value codes, but probably no other data entry program accepts .a in a numeric field. (See section 6.2 for more information about entering data.) When entering data, you might choose the codes –1 to –3 (provided, of course, that they could not be valid codes) and let Stata recode them:

```
. recode _all (-1=.)(-2=.a)(-3=.b)
```

mvdecode (see [D] **mvencode**) does essentially the same thing:

```
. mvdecode _all, mv(-1=. \ -2=.a \ -3=.b)
```

If you need to export data to another program that does not understand Stata's missing value codes, the reverse process could be performed:

```
. recode _all (.=-1)(.a=-2)(.b=-3)
```

However, mvencode is safer because it will refuse to recode to a value that already exists in the dataset:

```
. mvencode _all, mv(.=-1 \ .a=-2 \ .b=-3)
```

Precautions with missing values

You need not bother about the actual numerical values behind the missing values, but you need to know the logic to avoid mistakes. Missing values are high-end numbers; the ordering is

All valid numbers $< . < .a < .b < \cdots < .z$

Calculations involving one or more missing values lead to a missing result, and missing values are omitted from analyses, but the situation is different for logical expressions. The expression age>65 is true for an observation with missing age. Stata's behavior is predictable once you make this clear to yourself, but a warning is warranted:

WARNING! Missing values in logical expressions.

The following command initially surprised me by listing all whose ages were greater than 65 *and* those with missing age:

```
. list id age if age > 65
```

Technically, a missing value is larger than any valid number, which means that the expression age > 65 is true if age is missing values. To exclude the missing values, type

```
. list id age if age > 65 & age < .
```

To list the missing values only, including user-defined missing values, type

```
. list id age if age >=.
```

or

```
. list id age if missing(age)
```

5.4   Storage types and precision

Numeric variables can be integers (no decimals) and floating point numbers (with decimals). Integers come in three sizes: byte, int, and long; floating point numbers come in two sizes: float and double (double precision). Calculations are performed in double precision, but the default storage type of the result is float, as a compromise between precision and storage use. Read more in [U] **12.2.2 Numeric storage types**.

Variable type	Storage type	Bytes	Precision (digits)	Approx. range
Integer	byte	1	2	±100
	int	2	4	$\pm32,000$
	long	4	9	$\pm2\times10^9$
Floating point	float	4	7	$\pm10^{36}$
	double	8	16	$\pm10^{308}$

With large numbers, you may have problems with precision, as demonstrated in the following example:

```
. clear
. set obs 1                              Generate an empty observation
. generate xfloat=999999^2               A float (4-byte) variable
. generate double xdouble=999999^2       A double (8-byte) variable
. generate long xlong=999999^2           A long (4-byte) integer
. format xfloat-xlong %12.0f             Define display format
. list, clean
            xfloat       xdouble    xlong
   1.  999998029824   999998000001        .
```

xdouble shows the correct result; it is defined to be double precision. xfloat has the default float storage type; it is correct up to the first seven digits only. xlong is a long integer with a maximum of nine digits, too few for the result, which becomes missing.

You can see the storage types for the variables in a dataset with describe:

```
. describe
Contains data
  obs:            1
  vars:           3
  size:          20  (99.9% of memory free)

                storage  display    value
variable name   type     format     label      variable label

xfloat          float    %12.0f
xdouble         double   %12.0f
xlong           long     %12.0f

Sorted by:
    Note:  dataset has changed since last saved
```

The following gives another illustration of the phenomenon:

```
. clear
. set obs 1                      Create an empty observation
. gen xf = 1/7                   xf is float; 1/7 is double
. gen double xd = 1/7           xd is double; 1/7 is double
. list if xf == 1/7, clean
       (nothing happened)       xf (float) is not equal to 1/7 (double)
. list if xd == 1/7, clean      xd (double) is equal to 1/7 (double)
             xf         xd
   1.    .1428571   .1428571
```

Although we generated xf=1/7, the relational expression xf==1/7 was not true. xf is a float (4 bytes), while 1/7 during calculation is a double (8 bytes), and because of precision problems, xf and 1/7 were not equal. For the double-precision xd, the expression xd==1/7 was true. The expression xf==float(1/7) would be true, too.

The default float storage type uses 4 bytes per variable per observation, but variables often take small integer values only; they can be stored as a byte storage type. The command

```
. compress
```

finds the smallest possible storage type for each variable, which can substantially reduce memory requirements without compromising precision; see section 5.7 on memory considerations.

5.5 Date variables

Dates are numeric variables. The internal value is the number of days since 1 January 1960; the value of dates before that is negative. Date variables can be displayed in many different ways. See [U] **24 Dealing with dates**.

Date formats

Date formats are described in [U] **12.5.3 Date formats**. Format specifications start with %d. Specifying %d only is equivalent to %dD1CY, displaying a date as 19oct1993. To display this date as 19.10.1993, you would specify the format %dD.N.CY (D for day, N for numeric month, C for century, Y for two-digit year). To display it as 10/19/1993, you would type %dN/D/CY:

```
. clear
. set obs 1
. generate d1=12345
. generate d2=d1
. generate d3=d1
. generate d4=d1
. format d2 %d
. format d3 %dD.N.CY
. format d4 %dN/D/CY
. list, clean

          d1          d2          d3          d4
   1.   12345   19oct1993   19.10.1993   10/19/1993
```

Generating date variables

The numeric value of a date can be calculated from three variables—month, day, year (in that sequence)—and be formatted to be displayed as a date:

```
. generate bdate = mdy(bm,bd,by)
. format bdate %d
```

A date written as a string variable (sbdate) can be translated to a date variable:

```
. generate bdate = date(sbdate,"dmy")    "dmy" defines the sequence
. format bdate %dD.N.CY
```

The date() function understands many input formats: "17jan2001", "17/1/2001", "17.1.2001", "17 01 2001", but not "17012001". However, todate, a user-written command located at the SSC archives, handles this situation; install it by typing

```
. ssc install todate
```

Another command that might be useful in this context is nsplit, which can isolate selected digits from a numeric variable; you can install it by typing

```
. ssc install nsplit
```

In general, enter and display four-digit years to avoid ambiguity on the century. If you received data with two-digit years, you can make sure that they are interpreted as lying between, e.g., 1910 and 2010:

```
. generate bdate = date(sbdate,"dmy",2010)
```

Calculations with dates

You can calculate the length of a time interval as the difference in days between the last and the first date by typing

```
. generate days = date2 - date1
```

To express the length of a time interval in years, you must divide by 365.25:

```
. generate years = (date2 - date1)/365.25
```

You may extract day, month, and year from a date variable (bdate) by typing the following:

```
. generate bday = day(bdate)
. generate bmonth = month(bdate)
. generate byear = year(bdate)
```

Including time of day in calculations

Stata's date variables operate in days and do not include shorter intervals, such as hours, minutes, and seconds. But imagine that you observe patients (or mice, or petri dishes) and want to study intervals of hours, minutes, or seconds, and maybe even intervals spanning across midnight.

There are several user-written functions to egen (see section 8.3) in the egenmore package; you can install it by typing

```
. ssc install egenmore
```

The egenmore functions used below are

hms()   counting seconds since last midnight from the arguments h m s.

dhms()   calculating fractional date; the fractional part expresses the proportion of 24 hours since last midnight. Arguments (date h m s). The result is stored as double precision.

tod()   (time of day) making a string variable in the form hh:mm:ss from the number of seconds elapsed since last midnight.

```
. clear
. set obs 1
. generate x = mdy(5,6,1999)                   Generate a date (6 May 1999)
. generate date = x                            Make a copy of the date
. format date %d                               Define date format
. egen secs = hms(11 27 15)                    Seconds since midnight for 11:27:15
. egen datetime = dhms(date 11 27 15)          Fractional date, unit days (double
                                                   precision)
. generate str sdate = string(date, %d)        String variable for date in general
                                                   date format
. egen stime = tod(secs)                       String variable for time of day in the
                                                   form hh:mm:ss
. generate str sdatetime=sdate+" "+stime   Combine the two string variables,
                                                   displaying date and time
. list, clean
        x      date    secs    datetime     sdate    stime          sdatetime
  1.  14370  06may1999  41235   14370.477  06may1999  11:27:15  06may1999 11:27:15
```

The two important variables created are the double-precision numeric variable datetime, to be used for calculating time intervals, and sdatetime, a string variable displaying the date and time in a legible format. datetime's unit is days; to express an interval in hours, multiply by 24, etc.

5.6   String variables

Throughout this text, I have demonstrated the use of numeric variables, but Stata also handles string (text) variables. It is almost always easier and more flexible to use numeric variables, but sometimes you might need string variables. Read more in [U] **12.4 Strings** and [U] **23 Dealing with strings**. Read about string functions in [D] **functions**.

String values must be enclosed in quotes:

```
. replace ph=45 if nation == "Danish"
```

Because of case sensitivity, "Danish", "danish", and "DANISH" are different string values.

A string can include any character and numbers; however, number strings are not interpreted by their numeric value, just as a sequence of characters. Strings are sorted in dictionary sequence; however, all uppercase letters come before lowercase, numbers come before letters, and spaces or blanks come before anything else. This principle also applies to relations: " " < "12" < "2" < "A" < "AA" < "Z" < "a".

Do not confuse string variables with value labels for numeric variables. When you list observations without the nolabel option, the listed labels look the same as a string variable, but they are not; use describe to see the variable type. In the Data Editor, string variables are displayed in red, and value labels are in blue.

String formats

%10s displays a 10-character string, right-justified; %-10s displays it left-justified, for example,

```
. format patid %10s
```

Reading string variables into Stata

In the commands that read ASCII data (see section 6.4), the default data type is numeric, and string variables must be declared in the input command. str5 means a five-character text string:

```
. infix id 1-4 str5 icd10 5-9 using "a.txt"
```

Generating new string variables

The first time a string variable is defined, it can, but need not, be declared by its length (str10)

```
. generate str10 nation = "Danish" if ph==45
```

and this will work too:

```
. generate nation = "Danish" if ph==45
```

Conversion between string and numeric variables

Numeric strings to numbers

If a 10-digit number is stored in idstr (type string), no calculations can be performed. You could convert it to the numeric variable idnum by typing

```
. generate double idnum = real(idstr)
. format idnum %010.0f
```

idnum is a 10-digit number and must be declared `double` for sufficient precision (see section 5.4). The leading zero in the format descriptor displays leading zeros, if any.

Another possibility is `destring` (see [D] **destring**), which automatically stores `idnum` as a `double` if needed:

```
. destring idstr, generate(idnum)
. format idnum %010.0f
```

Nonnumeric strings to numbers

If a string variable `sex` were coded as "M" and "F", you could convert it to a numeric variable `gender` (with the original string codes as value labels) by typing

```
. encode sex, generate(gender)
```

encode will assign numeric codes in the string variable's alphabetic order. See [D] **encode**. You may, however, determine which strings get which codes by defining the value labels first:

```
. label define sexlbl 1 "M" 2 "F"
. encode sex, generate(gender) label(sexlbl)
```

Numbers to strings

You want to convert the numeric variable `idnum` to a string variable `idstr`. If you want any leading zeros to be included in the string, specify the format `"%010.0f"`:

```
. generate idstr = string(idnum, "%010.0f")
```

Another possibility is `tostring` (see [D] **destring**):

```
. tostring idnum, generate(idstr) format(%010.0f)
```

String manipulations

Strings can be added (concatenated) by typing +:

```
. clear
. set obs 1                              Generate empty observation
. generate svar3 = "abc"                 Generate a 3-character string
. generate svar2 = "de"                  Generate a 2-character string
. generate svar5 = svar3 + svar2         Add the strings
. list, clean

        svar3   svar2   svar5
  1.      abc      de   abcde
```

You can isolate part of a string variable by the substr() function. The arguments are source string, start position, and length. In the following, a3 will be characters 2–4 of svar5:

```
. generate a3 = substr(svar5,2,3)
. list, clean
          svar3   svar2   svar5   a3
     1.     abc      de   abcde  bcd
```

The upper() function converts lowercase to uppercase characters; the lower() function does the opposite. Imagine that ICD-10 codes had been entered inconsistently, with the same code sometimes as E10.1 and sometimes as e10.1. These are different strings, and you want them to be the same (E10.1):

```
. replace dx = upper(dx)
```

Handling complex strings, e.g., ICD-10 codes

In the International Classification of Diseases, 10th Revision (ICD-10) system, all codes are a combination of letters and numbers (e.g., E10.1 for insulin-demanding diabetes with ketoacidosis). This format is probably convenient for the person coding diagnoses (an important consideration), but for data management, it is inconvenient. I suggest splitting a five-character ICD-10 string variable (scode) into a one-character string variable (scode1) and a four-digit numeric variable (ncode4) by typing

```
. generate str1 scode1 = substr(scode,1,1)
. generate ncode4 = real(substr(scode,2,4))
. format ncode4 %4.1f
```

We obtained two variables: the string variable scode1 with 26 values (A–Z) and a numeric variable ncode4 (0.0–99.9). Now you can identify diabetes (E10.0–E14.9) by typing

```
. generate diab = 0
. replace diab = 1 if scode1=="E" & ncode4>=10 & ncode4<15
```

If you received ASCII data, you could have obtained the same result by letting the infix command read the same data twice as different types:

```
. infix id 1-4 str5 scode 5-9 str1 scode1 5 ncode4 6-9 using
> "list1.txt"
```

You could also have identified the diabetics this way:

```
. replace diab = 1 if scode >= "E10" & scode < "E15"
```

Another example: say that you received raw information from a hospital discharge register, where all ICD-10 codes had a D prefix, code lengths varied, and the decimal period was not included:

```
. list in 1/3
```

	diag
1.	DI73
2.	DI739
3.	DI739A

To reformat the codes to a conventional format, you could use the `substr()` function. `substr(diag,5,.)` means from character 5 to the end, and `%-6s` left-justified the string:

```
. generate diag1=substr(diag,2,3) + "." + substr(diag,5,.)
. format diag1 %-6s
. list in 1/3
```

	diag	diag1
1.	DI73	I73.
2.	DI739	I73.9
3.	DI739A	I73.9A

5.7   Memory considerations

In Intercooled Stata, a dataset can have a maximum of 2,047 variables (Stata/SE: 32,766). Stata keeps the entire dataset in memory, and the number of observations is limited by the memory allocated. The memory must be allocated before you load data into memory.

If the memory allocated is insufficient, you get the message:

```
no room to add more observations
```

You may increase the current memory (e.g., to 25 MB) by typing

```
. clear
. set memory 25m [, permanently]
```

You can see the amount of used and free memory by typing

```
. memory
```

If you allocate too much memory to Stata, you may make it slow down rather than improve its performance. So do not increase the memory allocated more than needed. You can read more in [D] **memory** and [U] **6 Setting the size of memory**.

compress

See [D] **compress**. To reduce the physical size and memory requirements of your dataset, Stata can determine the smallest storage type needed for each variable (see section 5.4), and you can safely type

```
. compress
```

and save the data again (`save, replace`). This step may reduce the memory needed by up to 80%.

Handling huge datasets

If you are handling a huge dataset, you may consider working on a subset of variables. Most often, you do not make analyses using all variables:

```
. use var1-var27 using hugeset.dta
```

You may consider increasing your computer's RAM (not expensive). For instance, with 512 MB of RAM, you could `set memory 400m` for Stata, and this allocation would fit very large datasets, e.g., a million observations with 100 variables. Stata/SE can handle up to 32,766 variables, but memory restrictions otherwise do not differ from those of Intercooled Stata. Thirty-two-bit processors cannot handle more than 2 GB of RAM, but with the new 64-bit processors, the amount is virtually infinite. To benefit from this increase, you must also purchase a 64-bit Stata version; ask StataCorp or your Stata distributor.

You might want to `compress` a huge dataset, but you cannot load it because of its large size. Try to read one part of the data, compress and save, read the next part of the data, compress and save, etc., and finally combine (`append`) the partial datasets (see section 9.4).

```
——————————— gen_aacomp.do ———————————
* gen_aacomp.do

cd C:\docs\proj1

use in 1/10000 using aa.dta, clear
compress
save aa1.dta

use in 10001/20000 using aa.dta, clear
compress
save aa2.dta

use in 20001/30000 using aa.dta, clear
compress

append using aa1.dta
append using aa2.dta
save aacomp.dta
```

If you encounter problems, carefully read [D] **memory**. Also read the FAQs on memory requirements for Windows (http://www.stata.com/support/faqs/win/); there are similar FAQs for other platforms.

6 Getting data in and out of Stata

6.1 Opening and saving Stata data

Precautions

When you open (use) a Stata dataset, you copy the contents of a disk file to the computer's memory (RAM). You can do any manipulation with the version in memory; it does not affect the contents of the disk file until you copy the version in memory back to the disk (save). It is like working with a word processor; you can write anything, but if you don't save the text before exiting, it has no permanent effect.

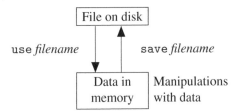

This is how most of us use a word processor. But have you ever, by mistake, overwritten good text with something else? (I have.) When it comes to your own data, collected at high expense, the cost of such a mistake may be high in terms of hours of work, or—worse—data loss or erroneous results. I strongly recommend the following principles:

- If you did not modify your data in memory, there is no point in saving them again.
- If you made modifications worth saving, save the revised data with a new filename, to avoid overwriting the original data. You might have made mistakes, and overwriting existing data might destroy valuable information.
- Make modifications worth saving with a do-file, including the initial use command, the modifying commands, and the final save command. This do-file documents what you did, and if you made any errors, you can correct the do-file and run it again.

- To avoid mistakes, specify the full file path when using and saving files. This can be done in two ways

      . cd C:\docs\proj1
      . use a1.dta
      . save a2.dta

  or

      . use C:\docs\proj1\a1.dta
      . save C:\docs\proj1\a2.dta

Read more about such precautions in chapter 18. The principle can be illustrated like this:

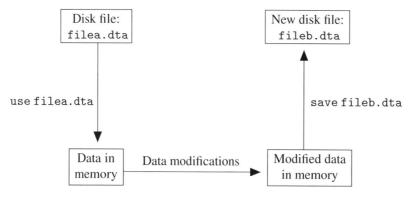

Defining the file path

Any survivors from the DOS era will recognize these commands, described in [D] **cd** and [D] **mkdir**.

cd stands for change directory. Instead of specifying the full path in the use and save commands, you could do it with cd by typing

      . cd C:\docs\proj1
      . use a1.dta
          (modifications to the data in memory)
      . save a2.dta

cd defines the working directory; its name is displayed in the lower-left corner of Stata's main window. You can also see it with the cd command. cd .. (space between cd and ..) moves up one directory. mkdir (make directory) creates a new directory. A sequence of commands could return the following output:

```
. cd                              Display current directory
C:\docs
. cd proj2                        Change to the proj2 subdirectory
C:\docs\proj2
. use a1.dta                      Use a1.dta in current directory
  (commands modifying data)
. save a2.dta                     Save a2.dta in current directory
file a2.dta saved
. cd ..                           Move up one directory level
C:\docs
. mkdir proj3                     Create new subdirectory proj3
```

If you use this method to define the file path, by all means include the cd command with the full path in every do-file; otherwise, the file location is undefined, with the risk of major mistakes.

use

The use command is documented in [D] **use**.

Copy an existing Stata dataset from disk to memory by typing

```
. cd C:\docs\proj1
. use a1.dta
```

or, alternatively

```
. use C:\docs\proj1\a1.dta
```

If there are data in memory, use will be rejected unless you specify the clear option. You may also issue the clear command before the use command to delete the data in memory

```
. use a1.dta, clear
```

or

```
. clear
. use a1.dta
```

Instead of typing the use command, you may click the 📂 ▾ button or select Open from the File menu.

If you want to use only observations that meet a certain condition, type

```
. use a1.dta if sex==1
```

If you want only the first 100 observations, type

```
. use a1.dta in 1/100
```

If you want to work with a subset of variables, type

```
. use age sex q1-q17 using a1.dta
```

In this book, you will meet two special use commands:

```
. sysuse auto.dta        Use a dataset that is part of your Stata installation
. webuse lbw.dta         Use a dataset available over the Internet
```

save

The save command is documented in [D] **save**.

Save the data in memory to a disk file by typing

```
. cd C:\docs\proj1
. save a2.dta
```

or, alternatively

```
. save C:\docs\proj1\a2.dta
```

If you already have saved a file with this name, you will need to use the replace option. This measure is a safeguard against destroying your data on disk: *use the* replace *option only if you really want to overwrite data.* A typical situation: you are developing a do-file ending with a save command; you need to modify your first attempts so you need to use the replace option:

```
. save a2.dta, replace
```

save does not allow restrictions to a subset of observations or variables; use the keep command (see section 9.2) if that is what you want by typing

```
. keep age sex q1-q17
. save a2.dta, replace
```

Instead of typing the save command, you can click the 💾 button or select Save As from the File menu.

6.2   Entering data

In [U] **21 Inputting data** and [D] **infile**, you will find an overview of the different ways to enter data.

The input command

For small datasets, you can define the variables with the `input` command and enter the values. Finish the input with `end`. It can be done interactively from the command line or in a do-file. See [D] **input**, and see more examples in section 11.8 (*Graph examples*).

```
. clear
. input case expose pop
    0 0 100
    0 1 30
    1 0 23
    1 1 21
    end
```

Using Stata's Data Editor to enter data

You may use Stata's Data Editor to enter data in a spreadsheet format; for a tutorial, see the *Getting Started* manual. If you are entering many data, however, you may not want to use the spreadsheet format, and you should use a specialized program for data entry; see below.

Using a data entry program

If you are going to enter more than a few data, you will benefit from a specialized program for data entry. A good program for entering data should

- Enable you to set up a screen resembling, for example, a questionnaire page. This makes data entry easier and reduces the risk of errors (entering the right information in the wrong place).
- Check the validity of the data entered (checking that the data entered are within defined ranges).
- Enable you to enter data twice and compare the two files.
- Allow you to export data to the statistical program you use.

One such program is EpiData, which can be downloaded at no cost. It is easy to learn and easy to install. It can export data to Stata, SAS, SPSS, and spreadsheets. In section 18.3, I give some more advice on entering data.

At the author's web site, you will find a short description of EpiData and instructions on obtaining it and using it to produce Stata datasets; see *Other supplementary materials provided by the author* at http://www.stata-press.com/books/ishr.html.

6.3   Reading ASCII data

On decimal periods and commas

Stata cannot read or write ASCII data with decimal commas, regardless of the Windows settings. The Stata command `set dp comma` affects how values are displayed, not how they are written to or read from ASCII files.

If your computer displays decimal commas, I suggest that you change the Windows settings by selecting

[Start] ▷ Settings ▷ Control Panel ▷ Regional and Language Options

Here you can choose a country that uses decimal periods.

If you received an ASCII file with decimal commas from someone else, you could use a text editor to replace the commas with periods—but if the file has text strings including commas you then create another problem. Another way around the problem, if the file is tab-delimited or semicolon-delimited (see below), is to

1. Change the Windows settings to use decimal commas.

2. Import the text file to a spreadsheet program such as Excel.

3. Change the Windows settings to use decimal periods.

4. Export data as a tab-delimited text file; it now has decimal periods.

Reading tab- or comma-separated data

For more information about reading tab- or comma-separated data, see [D] **insheet**. In tab-separated data, the tab character, here displayed as <T>, separates the values. A tab-separated ASCII file is created, for example, if you save an Excel worksheet as a text (`.txt`) file. If row 1 has variable names, Stata will figure this out and use them, but the variable names must follow Stata's rules (no spaces or special characters).

In this and the following examples, the value of `type` in observation 2 is missing:

```
id <T> type <T> sold <T> price
1 <T> 2 <T> 47 <T> 51.23
2 <T> <T> 793 <T> 199.70
```

You can read a tab-separated ASCII file with variable names in row 1 by typing the command

```
. insheet using a.txt, tab
```

In comma-separated data, commas separate the values:

```
1,2,47,51.23
2,,793,199.70
```

If you have a comma-separated file without variable names in row 1, you would use the command

> . insheet id type sold price using a.txt, comma

and with any other separator (here a semicolon), you would use

> . insheet id type sold price using a.txt, delimit(";")

insheet assumes that all data belonging to one observation are in one line.

Reading free-format data

See [D] **infile (free format)** for detail on reading free-format data. In free-format data, commas or blank spaces separate the values:

```
1 2 47 51.23
2 .   793 199.70
```

The command for reading such data is

> . infile id type sold price using a.txt

infile does not assume that data belonging to one observation are in one line. infile considers the following data to be the same as the data above:

```
1 2 47 51.23 2 .   793 199.70
```

Reading fixed-format data

For detailed information about reading fixed-format data, see [D] **infix (fixed format)**. In fixed-format data, the information on each variable is determined by the position in the line; these positions are defined in the infix command. The blank type in observation 2 will be read as missing.

```
12 47 51.23
2 793199.70
```

The command for reading these data is

> . infix id 1 type 2 sold 3-5 price 6-11 using a.txt

Fixed-format data can also be read by infile; to do this, you must create a dictionary file, specifying variable names and positions, etc. See [D] **infile (fixed format)**.

6.4   Exchanging data with other programs

> **Take care:** Translation between programs may go wrong, so you should carefully
> compare the output from Stata's summarize and, e.g., SPSS's DESCRIPTIVES and
> compare the number of valid values for each variable and the minimum and maximum
> values. Be especially careful with missing values and date variables.

Translation programs

If you use more than one statistical program, or if you are switching from another program
to Stata, you will need a program to translate your data. One such translation program is
Stat/Transfer (available from Circle Systems). Variable names, variables, and value labels are
transferred as part of the data. Stat/Transfer 7 and 8 translate Stata 8 and Stata 9 files, but
Stat/Transfer 6 does not. To create a Stata dataset for conversion by Stat/Transfer 6, type

```
. saveold alfa.dta
```

Transferring data to Excel and other spreadsheets

Stata can save a dataset in XML format, which can be read by Excel; see [D] **xmlsave**:

```
. sysuse auto.dta
(1978 Automobile Data)
. xmlsave auto.xml, doctype(excel)
```

Before Stata 9, a more traditional method was needed (and it still works): create a tab-
separated file with variable names in the first row to be read by a spreadsheet; see [D] **outsheet**:

```
. outsheet [varlist] using alfa.txt, nolabel
```

In Excel, open the file as a text file, and follow the instructions. Variable names, but not
labels, are transferred. A similar file without variable names in the first row is created by typing

```
. outsheet [varlist] using alfa.txt, nolabel nonames
```

If you want to write the data to a comma-separated ASCII file, use the command (see [D] **out-
file**)

```
. outfile [varlist] using alfa.txt, nolabel comma
```

Make sure you set your Windows international settings to use decimal periods; see section 6.3.

Rather than looking up the commands, you might prefer to use the menu system. Start by
selecting

> File ▷ Export

Reading spreadsheet data

Stata can read a dataset in XML format, which could be created by Excel; see [D] **xmlsave**. The `firstrow` option means that the first row in the spreadsheet should be interpreted as variable names:

```
. xmluse auto.xml, doctype(excel) sheet("Sheet1") firstrow
```

For this to work, the Excel worksheet must have a simple rectangular structure with variable names in the first row. Also, the variable names must fulfill Stata's requirements: they must be unique and not include spaces or special characters.

Prior to Stata 9, a more traditional method was needed (and it still works); see [D] **insheet**. Many packages can create Excel data, and most can create text files like those created by Stata's `outsheet` command. In Excel, you save a tab-separated text file; Stata reads it by typing

```
. insheet using a.txt, tab
```

Rather than looking up the commands, you might prefer to use the menu system; select

File ▷ Import

Copying and pasting between a spreadsheet and Stata's Data Editor

Copying and pasting between a spreadsheet and Stata's Data Editor works almost by intuition. But beware that the the risk of errors is rather high, and you may encounter problems with variable types, for example, that a variable that should be numeric is converted to a string variable. Again, Windows should be set to display decimal periods; otherwise, it will not work right.

There is an FAQ about it by N. J. Cox: *How do I get information from Excel into Stata?* at http://www.stata.com/support/faqs/data/newexcel.html.

ODBC: Open DataBase Connectivity

`odbc` allows Stata to load data from ODBC sources, such as certain databases. You can read more in [D] **odbc**.

Translation between SAS and Stata using FDA file formats

`fdasave` and `fdause` convert datasets to and from the FDA's (U.S. Food and Drug Administration) SAS format for new drug and device applications. The primary intent of these commands is to assist people making submissions to the FDA, but the commands are general enough to use in transferring data between SAS and Stata. Read more in [D] **fdasave**.

7 Documentation commands

Documentation commands let you add explanatory text to your data. A dataset label gives you descriptive information when you open the dataset. Variable labels and value labels add explanatory text to output from analyses.

You do not need documentation commands to analyze data, but using them will help make your output legible and reduce the risk of errors when interpreting the output.

7.1 Labels

You can read more about labels in [D] **label**.

Dataset label

You can give a short description of your data to be displayed every time you open (use) data by typing

```
. label data "Fertility data Denmark 1997-99. ver 2.5, 19sep2002"
```

Include the creation date to be sure of which version you are analyzing.

Variable labels

You can attach explanatory text to a variable name:

```
. label variable q6 "Ever itchy skin rash?"
```

Use informative labels, but make them short; long variable labels are often abbreviated in output.

Value labels

You can attach explanatory text to each code for a categorical variable. This is a two-step procedure. First, define the label (using double quotes around text with embedded blanks):

```
. label define sexlbl  1 male  2 female  9 "sex unknown"
```

Next associate the label sexlbl with the variable sex:

```
. label values sex sexlbl
```

Use informative labels, but make them short; value labels are often abbreviated to 12 characters in output.

Most often, you will use the same name for a variable and its label

```
. label define sex  1 male  2 female
. label values sex sex
```

but defining the label enables you to reuse it:

```
. label define yesno  1 yes  2 no
. label values q1 yesno
. label values q2 yesno
. ...
```

If you want to modify a label definition or add new labels, use the `modify` option:

```
. label define sexlbl 9 "unknown sex", modify
```

In output, Stata displays either the value labels or the codes (the `nolabel` option). You often need to see them both, however, to avoid mistakes. You can do so by including the codes in the labels using the `numlabel` command; see [D] **labelbook**.

```
. numlabel [lblname-list], add
```

See label definitions

`codebook` with the `compact` option displays the variable labels and other summary information about the variables. This command is most useful for obtaining an overview of a dataset:

```
. sysuse auto.dta, clear
(1978 Automobile Data)

. codebook, compact
```

Variable	Obs	Unique	Mean	Min	Max	Label
make	74	74	.	.	.	Make and Model
price	74	74	6165.257	3291	15906	Price
mpg	74	21	21.2973	12	41	Mileage (mpg)
rep78	69	5	3.405797	1	5	Repair Record 1978
headroom	74	8	2.993243	1.5	5	Headroom (in.)
trunk	74	18	13.75676	5	23	Trunk space (cu. ft.)
weight	74	64	3019.459	1760	4840	Weight (lbs.)
length	74	47	187.9324	142	233	Length (in.)
turn	74	18	39.64865	31	51	Turn Circle (ft.)
displacement	74	31	197.2973	79	425	Displacement (cu. in.)
gear_ratio	74	36	3.014865	2.19	3.89	Gear Ratio
foreign	74	2	.2972973	0	1	Car type

Typing `describe` gives you more information on formats and labels:

```
. describe
Contains data from C:\Stata\ado\base/a/auto.dta
  obs:            74                          1978 Automobile Data
  vars:           12                          13 Apr 2005 17:45
  size:        3,478 (99.9% of memory free)   (_dta has notes)

                 storage  display   value
variable name    type     format    label    variable label

make             str18    %-18s               Make and Model
price            int      %8.0gc              Price
mpg              int      %8.0g               Mileage (mpg)
   (output omitted)
foreign          byte     %8.0g     origin    Car type
```

One variable (foreign) also has value labels (origin), which you can list by typing

```
. label list
    origin:
           0 Domestic
           1 Foreign
```

Typing labelbook gives you more details about the labels; see [D] **labelbook**.

Typing codebook (without the compact option) gives you a lot of information for each variable; see section 10.1.

Notes

You may add notes to your dataset; see [D] **notes**:

```
. notes: 19oct2000. Corrections made after proof-reading
```

and to single variables:

```
. notes age: 20oct2000. Ages > 120 and < 0 recoded to missing
```

The notes are stored in the dataset; you can display them by typing

```
. notes
```

Notes are cumulative; old notes are not discarded, but you can drop notes by the notes drop command (see [D] **notes**).

7.2 Working with labels: an example

In the auto.dta dataset, foreign is a strange variable name; I want to change it to origin. The variable label is "Car type"; I think "Country of origin" is a better choice. And living outside the United States, I want the value labels "Domestic" and "Foreign" replaced by "U.S." and "Other".

For this example, I begin by renaming the variable and removing the current labels:

```
. sysuse auto.dta
(1978 Automobile Data)
. rename foreign origin      See section 9.3
. label variable origin      Remove any variable label
. label drop origin          Drop value label origin
```

With no labels defined, a simple frequency table looks like this:

```
. tab1 origin

-> tabulation of origin
     origin │      Freq.      Percent          Cum.
────────────┼───────────────────────────────────────
          0 │         52        70.27         70.27
          1 │         22        29.73        100.00
────────────┼───────────────────────────────────────
      Total │         74       100.00
```

This display is not very informative; you cannot see the meaning of origin or the meaning of the codes 0 and 1. Defining variable and value labels is helpful:

```
. label variable origin "Country of origin"
. label define origin 0 "U.S." 1 "Other"
. label values origin origin
. tab1 origin

-> tabulation of origin
 Country of │
     origin │      Freq.      Percent          Cum.
────────────┼───────────────────────────────────────
       U.S. │         52        70.27         70.27
      Other │         22        29.73        100.00
────────────┼───────────────────────────────────────
      Total │         74       100.00
```

Now the table displays explanatory text (Country of origin) and the meaning of the codes (U.S., Other) rather than the codes themselves (0, 1). This clarification makes the table easier to read and reduces the risk of mistakes. It would, however, be useful to see the codes and the value labels at the same time; you can do this by using the numlabel command:

```
. numlabel, add
. tab1 origin

-> tabulation of origin
 Country of │
     origin │      Freq.      Percent          Cum.
────────────┼───────────────────────────────────────
    0. U.S. │         52        70.27         70.27
   1. Other │         22        29.73        100.00
────────────┼───────────────────────────────────────
      Total │         74       100.00
```

Now you have all the information you need: you have defined the `origin` variable (Country of origin) and its codes (0: U.S.; 1: Other). Seeing the codes and the value labels together is useful, among other reasons because the `if` qualifier needs the code, not the value label:

```
. summarize if origin == "U.S."
type mismatch
r(109);
```

Stata did not understand your intent; the `type mismatch` message is due to a mismatch between the numeric variable `origin` and the string "`U.S.`". You must ask for the code, not the label:

```
. summarize if origin == 0
```

In the example shown, you should include the commands in a do-file. This file differs a bit from what you saw before, but it has the same effect.

```
─────────────────────── gen_auto2.do ───────────────────────
* gen_auto2.do generates auto2.dta:  Revised labels

sysuse auto.dta, clear
rename foreign origin                       // Change variable name
label variable origin "Country of origin"   // Define variable label
label define origin 0 "U.S." 1 "Other", modify   // Define value labels
label values origin origin                  // and apply to variable
numlabel origin, add                        // Add codes to value labels
compress                                     // A good place to do this

cd C:\docs\ishr
save auto2.dta, replace                      // Save revised dataset
```

The variable and value label definition are now included in `auto2.dta`. Adding or modifying labels is a modification of the dataset, so you should use a do-file that generates a dataset with a new name.

Chapter 18 will give you more advice and some more tools for documenting your data. As you have already seen, I favor using sensible variable names, informative labels, and do-files with names that tell what they do (`gen_auto2.do` generates `auto2.dta`).

8   Calculations

Calculation commands generate new variables or modify the values of existing variables. This chapter concerns numeric variables; string manipulations were explained in section 5.6.

Operators and functions for calculations are shown in section 8.2; you can also read more in [D] **generate** and [U] **13 Functions and expressions**.

8.1   generate and replace

Generate a new variable by typing

```
. generate bmi = weight/(height^2)
```

If the target variable (bmi) already exists in the dataset, generate will be rejected, and you must replace bmi by typing

```
. replace bmi = weight/(height^2)
```

The distinction between generate and replace is a safeguard to prevent you from unintentionally overwriting existing data. generate is one of the few commands I abbreviate (to gen); replace cannot be abbreviated for reasons of safety.

Using the if qualifier

You can use the if qualifier to restrict the calculations to a subset of data. To do calculations for males only, type

```
. generate mbmi = 1.1*bmi if sex==1   This example is nonsense
. replace npreg = . if sex==1         N of pregnancies missing for males
                                           (question not asked)
```

Using the in qualifier

You can use the in qualifier to restrict the calculations to specific observations. This may be used, e.g., for corrections:

```
. replace weight = 87 in 227          Correction to observation 227
```

Using the by...: construct

You can use the by *varlist*: prefix when numbering observations:

> . by sex, sort: generate obsno = _n   Consecutive numbering within each sex
>   (example section 8.5)

Calculations involving missing values

If a calculation involves a missing value, the result will be missing; for the calculations above, bmi will be missing if height or weight is missing.

Calculations involving logical expressions

If we want to use a BMI value to classify people as obese (BMI$\geq$ 30) or not obese (BMI$<$ 30), we can do so in several ways. One way is to use recode (see section 8.4):

> . recode bmi (30/max=1)(min/30=0), generate(obese)

Another option is to do the following; be careful not to include missing BMIs as obese:

> . generate obese=0
> . replace obese=1 if bmi>=30
> . replace obese=. if bmi>=.

You can use one command to obtain the same results as the previous three: the right-hand side of a calculation can be a logical expression that can evaluate to 0 (meaning false) or 1 (meaning true):

> . generate obese = bmi>=30

The target variable (obese) takes the value 0 if bmi $<$ 30 and 1 if bmi $\geq$ 30. But take care: a missing value is a large number, and the expression will evaluate to true if bmi is missing. There are two ways to handle this problem; one is to let obese be false (i.e., 0) if bmi is missing:

> . generate obese = bmi>=30 & bmi<.

Another option (and usually a more consistent option) is to let obese be missing if bmi is missing:

> . generate obese = bmi>=30 if bmi<.

The three ways to handle a missing value in a logical expression are illustrated below:

> . generate obese1 = bmi>=30
> . generate obese2 = bmi>=30 & bmi<.
> . generate obese3 = bmi>=30 if bmi<.

```
. list bmi obese*, clean

     bmi  obese1  obese2  obese3
  1.  29       0       0       0
  2.  31       1       1       1
  3.   .       1       0       .
```

A variable can be evaluated as a logical expression; in the `auto.dta` dataset, the variable `foreign` takes the value 0 for domestic cars and 1 for foreign cars, and you can type

. **summarize if foreign**   Foreign cars (`foreign=1`)

. **summarize if !foreign**   Domestic cars (`foreign=0`)

The value 0 evaluates to false, whereas any other value, *including missing*, evaluates to true, so be careful: the expression `foreign` will evaluate to true for observations with `foreign` missing.

For an instructive FAQ by N. J. Cox, see *What is true and false in Stata?* at http://www.stata.com/support/faqs/data/trueorfalse.html.

Checking your results

When you have made any complex modifications, check to see if they worked as intended

. **list weight height bmi in 1/5**

or

. **browse weight height bmi in 1/5**

and check a few observations for correctness. Also type

. **summarize bmi**

and look at minimum and maximum values, applying your knowledge that BMI values less than 15 and more than 40 are unusual.

8.2   Operators and functions in calculations

Arithmetic operators

There are five arithmetic operators; see [U] **13 Functions and expressions**.

---

  ^   power

  *   multiplication

  /   division

  +   addition

  –   subtraction

The order of operations is as shown in the table; power comes before multiplication and division, which come before addition and subtraction:

```
. generate alcohol = beers + wines + spirits
. generate bmi = weight/(height^2)
```

The parentheses in the last command ensure that `height^2` is calculated before the division. Here, however, the parentheses are not necessary since power takes precedence over division—but they do not cause any harm.

```
. generate z = a+b/y
```

means the same as

```
. generate z = a+(b/y)
```

but is different from

```
. generate z = (a+b)/y
```

since division is performed before addition. When in doubt, use parentheses; they may also make the command more transparent to you. For transparency, you can also use spacing, but spacing does not change a Stata command, so

```
. generate z = a + b/y
```

means the same to Stata as

```
. generate z = a+b / y
```

Functions

Besides the operators shown, there are several functions available in Stata; see [D] **functions**. I show some examples with `generate`, some with `display` (see section 10.6), but they are the same functions. Examples:

Mathematical functions:

`. generate y=abs(x)`	Absolute value: $\lvert x \rvert$
`. gen y=exp(x)`	Exponential, e^x
`. gen y=ln(x)`	Natural logarithm
`. gen y=log10(x)`	Base 10 logarithm
`. gen y=sqrt(x)`	Square root
`. gen y=int(x)`	Integer part of x; $\mathtt{int(5.8)} = 5$; $\mathtt{int(-5.8)} = -5$
`. gen y=floor(x)`	Rounding down; $\mathtt{floor(-5.8)} = -6$
`. gen y=ceil(x)`	Rounding up; $\mathtt{ceil(5.8)} = 6$
`. gen y=round(x)`	Nearest integer; $\mathtt{round(5.8)} = 6$
`. gen y=round(x,0.25)`	$\mathtt{round(5.8,0.25)} = 5.75$

. gen y=mod(x1,x2)	Modulus; the remainder after dividing x1 by x2
. gen y=max(x1,...,xn)	Maximum value of arguments
. gen y=min(x1,...,xn)	Minimum value of arguments
. gen y=sum(x)	Cumulative sum from first to current observation
. gen y=sign(x)	Returns –1 if $x < 0$; 0 if $x = 0$, 1 if $x > 0$, . if x is missing

Statistical functions:

. display chi2tail(*df*, *chi2*)	chi2tail(1, 3.84) = 0.05
. display invchi2tail(*df*, *Pr*)	invchi2tail(1, 0.05) = 3.84
. display normal(*z*)	normal(-1.96) = 0.025
. display invnormal(*Pr*)	invnormal(0.025) = -1.96
. display ttail(*df*, *t*)	ttail(20, 2.09) = 0.025
. display invttail(*df*, *Pr*)	invttail(20, 0.025) = 2.09

_n, _N, and some other functions:

. gen y=_n	_n is the observation number
. gen y=_N	_N is the number of observations in the dataset
. gen y=cond(*exp*, *a*, *b*, *c*), e.g.,	
. gen y=cond(x>z,1,-1,.)	Returns *a* if *exp* is true, *b* if *exp* is false, *c* if *exp* is missing
. gen y=uniform()	Returns a random number in the range 0–1 (section 16.1)

There must be no space between the function name and the open parenthesis enclosing the arguments:

This is wrong:	. generate y=round (x)
This is right:	. generate y=round(x)

Look in [D] **functions** or use help functions to find many other functions, such as trigonometric functions:

```
. generate y = sin(x)
```

To see the online help for a function, include parentheses after the function name:

```
. help sin()
```

String functions are described in section 5.6, and date functions are covered in section 5.5.

8.3   Extended functions: egen

egen (extensions to generate) provides more functions; see [D] **egen**. egen has no alternative like replace, and if the target variable, e.g., meanage, already exists, you must choose another variable name or

```
. drop meanage
```

before resubmitting the egen command. Here are some examples:

Generating the same value for all observations

```
. egen meanage=mean(age)            Mean age across observations
. by sex: egen meanage=mean(age)    Mean age across observations, for each sex
. egen medage=median(age)           Median age across observations
. egen sumage=total(age)            Sum across all observations
. egen maxage=max(age)              Maximum value of age across observations
. egen minage=min(age)              Minimum value of age across observations
. egen validage=count(age)          Number of nonmissing age across observations
```

The above functions generate variables that are constant across the dataset (or across each subset defined by by...:); conceptually using one of these functions is like spreading the information from a summarize across the dataset. Missing values are excluded from the calculations.

Generating individual values for each observation (each row)

```
. egen qmin=rowmin(q1-q17)          Minimum value of q1-q17 for this observation
. egen qmax=rowmax(q1-q17)          Maximum value of q1-q17 for this observation
. egen qmean=rowmean(q1-q17)        Mean value of q1-q17 for this observation
. egen qsum=rowtotal(q1-q17)        Sum of q1-q17 for this observation
. egen qmiss=rowmiss(q1-q17)        Number of missing q1-q17 for this observation
. egen qvalid=rownonmiss(q1-q17)    Number of nonmissing   q1-q17 for this
                                      observation
```

For the first four of the above functions, any missing values are excluded from the analysis. If you want to calculate the mean if there are at least five nonmissing values, type

```
. egen qvalid = rownonmiss(q1-q17)
. egen qmean = rowmean(q1-q17) if qvalid > 4
```

Some of the above functions have cousins in the general Stata functions but are slightly different. egen's rowmax() function takes a variable list but no other arguments. Stata's max() function can take constants and variables, but not in variable list format:

```
. egen vmax = rowmax(v1-v5)           rowmax() takes a variable list
. egen vmax = rowmax(v1 v2 v3 v4 v5)  egen forbids commas between arguments
. generate vmax = max(v1,v2,v3,v4,v5) generate requires commas between
                                        arguments
. generate vmax = max(v1,v2,0)        max() also takes constant arguments
```

The group() function

The group() function lets you generate a new variable with all possible combinations of the categories of one or more variables. This may be useful when you want a stratified analysis with more than one variable defining the strata. If sex has two categories and race has three, racesex will get six categories:

```
. egen racesex = group(race sex), label
. cc low smoke, by(racesex)
```

See section 8.5 for an example of using group() to give numbers to patients who could have several hospital admissions.

The cut() function

The cut() function lets you create groups from a continuous variable; this is a convenient way to recode a continuous variable into intervals of equal width. The numeric list should include a large number (200); if it had not, ages 85 and older would have been recoded to missing. The code for an interval is its lower limit:

```
. egen agegr=cut(age), at(0 5(10)85 200)
```

age	agegr
$0 \leq \text{age} < 5$	0
$5 \leq \text{age} < 15$	5
$15 \leq \text{age} < 25$	15
$\ldots$	
$85 \leq \text{age} < 200$	85

With the label option, the value labels will be 0-, 5-, etc.; the codes themselves will be consecutive integers, starting at 0:

```
. egen agegr=cut(age), at(0 5(10)85 200) label
```

age	agegr	Value label
$0 \leq \text{age} < 5$	0	0-
$5 \leq \text{age} < 15$	1	5-
$15 \leq \text{age} < 25$	2	15-
$\ldots$		
$85 \leq \text{age} < 200$	9	85-

Another use of the `cut()` function is to create groups with approximately equal numbers of observations; here there are five groups:

```
. egen agegr=cut(age), group(5) label
```

I rarely use the `group()` option; I prefer to present groups with "natural" intervals, and the `at()` option (or `recode`; see section 8.4) lets me do that.

The egenmore functions

egen allows skilled and creative users to invent new, unofficial functions; `egenmore` is a library of such functions. You can install them by typing

```
. ssc install egenmore
```

An example is shown in section 5.5 (date variables).

8.4   Recoding variables

See [D] **recode** for details on recoding variables. `recode` is useful, for example, for modifying codes of a categorical variable:

```
. recode sex (0=2)        sex was F:0, M:1; now M:1, F:2
```

But be aware, first, that the rule not to overwrite original data was violated, and second, that the value labels no longer match the codes. A good solution, which creates a new variable (gender) and defines value labels at once, is to type

```
. recode sex (1=1 "male") (0=2 "female"), generate(gender)
. numlabel gender, add
. label variable gender "Sex of respondent"
```

If the target variable (gender) already exists, you will get an error message, so you must choose another variable name or type

```
. drop gender
```

before resubmitting the `recode` command.

Another option, of course, is to define value labels the standard way:

```
. recode sex (0=2), generate(gender)
. label define gender  1 male  2 female
. label values gender gender
. numlabel gender, add
. label variable gender "Sex of respondent"
```

The important point is that you should define labels at once when you create a new variable. It will never be easier than at that point; it will only be more difficult if you postpone it. If you do not create labels, the risk of making mistakes is high.

recode is also typically used to generate a new categorical variable (agegr) from a continuous variable (age). age is recorded in years, but with the precision of days, and I want to ensure that age 55.00 (at the birthday) goes to category 4:

```
. recode age (55/max=4)(35/55=3)(15/35=2)(min/15=1), generate(agegr)
```

The value 55 was specified in both the first and the second intervals, but the information was "taken" by the first. When recode intervals overlap, the first interval specified wins.

Again, labels for the new variable should be defined at once:

```
. recode age (55/max=4 "55+")(35/55=3 "35-54")(15/35=2 "15-34")
> (min/15=1 "-14"), generate(agegr)
. numlabel agegr, add
. label variable agegr "Age at admission, grouped"
```

Important: The generate() option creates a new variable with the recoded information. With

```
. recode age (55/max=4)(35/55=3)(15/35=2)(min/15=1)
```

age would be recoded into itself, meaning that the original information in age would be destroyed. You should never destroy primary information but rather create a new variable with the recoded information; the generate() option enables you to do that.

A continuous variable could also be grouped using egen's cut() function; see section 8.3.

If you made modifications of any complexity, check at once to see whether it worked as intended. To check the recoding of sex into gender, type

```
. tab2 sex gender
```

To check the recoding of age into agegr, type

```
. sort age
. list age agegr  [, nolabel]
```

or

```
. sort age
. browse age agegr [, nolabel]
```

The sorting makes it easy to concentrate on the critical ages (15, 35, 55). You can make it even easier by making a separator line when agegr changes:

```
. list age agegr, sepby(agegr)
```

Another useful method for checking a recode operation is to inspect a scatterplot (see chapter 11):

```
. twoway (scatter agegr age), xlabel(0 15 35 55, grid)
```

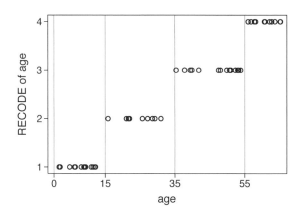

Figure 8.1: Using a scatterplot to check `recode`

Other `recode` examples:

`. recode x (2=0)`	Values not recoded left unchanged
`. recode x (2=0), generate(x2)`	Values not recoded transferred unchanged
`. recode x (2=0) if sex==1`	Observations not included (`sex !=1`) left unchanged
`. recode x (2=0) if sex==1, gen(x2)`	x2 set to missing if `sex !=1`
`. recode x (2=0) if sex==1, gen(x2) copyrest`	Values transferred unchanged if `sex !=1`
`. recode x (2=0)(1=1)(else=9) [, gen(x2)]`	Recode remaining values to 9
`. recode x (9=.)`	Recode 9 to system missing
`. recode x (.=9)`	Recode system missing to 9
`. recode x (missing=9)`	Recode any missing value to 9

8.5   Numbering observations

The variable age in the third observation can be referred to as `age[3]`; for more information, see [U] **13.7 Explicit subscripting**. The principle is

age	Current observation
age[_n]	Current observation
age[1]	First observation
age[_N]	Last observation
age[_n-1]	Previous (lag) observation
age[_n+1]	Next (lead) observation
age[27]	Observation 27

The following is a valid command:

```
. generate x = age[27]
```

This command sets x to the same value in all observations. However, explicit subscripting cannot take place to the left of the equal sign, and the following command is not valid:

```
. replace x[28] = 15
```

Instead type

```
. replace x = 15 in 28
```

Example: from a patient register you have information about hospital admissions, one or more per person, identified by patid (a 10-digit personal ID) and admdate (admission date). You want to construct the following variables: obsno (observation number), patno (study ID), admno (admission number), and admtot (patient's total number of admissions).

The do-file gen_patnumbers.do uses subscripting. With the by: construct, _n and _N apply to each subgroup, and typing

```
. by patid: generate admtot = _N
```

generates the total number of admissions for each patient.

(*Continued on next page*)

─────────────────── gen_patnumbers.do ───────────────────

```
* gen_patnumbers.do
cd C:\docs\ishr
use admissions.dta, clear

* Sort by patient and date of admission, and generate observation number
sort patid admdate
generate obsno = _n
label variable obsno "Observation number"

* Give each patient a number
egen patno = group(patid)
label variable patno "Patient number"

* Generate admission number and total admissions for each patient
by patid: generate admno = _n
label variable admno "Patient's admission number"
by patid: generate admtot = _N
label variable admtot "Patient's number of admissions"

save patnumbers.dta, replace
```

The result is shown here; it worked as intended:

```
. list in 1/7, sepby(patno)
```

	patid	admdate	obsno	patno	admno	admtot
1.	0605401234	01may1970	1	1	1	3
2.	0605401234	16may1970	2	1	2	3
3.	0605401234	04mar1971	3	1	3	3
4.	1705401234	22feb1970	4	2	1	1
5.	2705401235	01jan1970	5	3	1	1
6.	2805402345	29jan1970	6	4	1	2
7.	2805402345	14jul1970	7	4	2	2

Now the number of patients is displayed as the maximum by typing

    . summarize patno

To study first admissions, type

    . *anycommand* if admno==1

To study final admissions, type

    . *anycommand* if admno==admtot

And to see the distribution of the patients' number of admissions, type

    . tab1 admtot if admno==1

8.6 Exercises

8-1. Open the auto.dta dataset (sysuse auto.dta), and get an overview by typing codebook, compact.

All measurements are in U.S. units, but you are trying to get the results published in an international journal that requires the international metric units (e.g., meters, liters, kilograms). The following conversions apply:

US units		International units
1 inch	=	2.54 cm
1 foot	=	30.48 cm
1 mile	=	1,609 m
1 gallon	=	3.785 L
1 pound	=	0.454 kg

Generate new variables—with reasonable names, e.g., mweight for metric weight—describing the cars' performance in metric units (mileage expressed in km/L, etc.). Furnish the variables with relevant labels, and save a new dataset (the suggested name is metricauto.dta).

8-2. For the first few observations, examine whether the calculations are correct (list or browse in 1/5). (I recommend using list and making a printout; it is more efficient and less straining than looking at the screen).

8-3. Print a new codebook, compact table that includes both the old and the new variables.

8-4. Create a do-file that does steps 8-1 to 8-3. (Create a do-file from the Review window or the command log; see section 1.7). I recommend using the name gen_metricauto.do for the do-file that generates metricauto.dta. Check that the do-file works by running it.

8-5. Use `recode` to generate a new variable, `mweightgr`, grouped in 500-kg intervals. Put appropriate labels on `mweightgr`. Before deciding the intervals, see the minimum and maximum values of `mweight` (`codebook`, `compact` or `summarize`).

8-6. Check that the calculation of `mweightgr` worked as intended by using the following commands:

```
. sort mweight
. list mweight mweightgr, sepby(mweightgr)
```

What is the benefit of sorting before listing? What is the effect of the `sepby()` option? You might also try a scatterplot, such as the one in figure 8.1.

8-7. Make a simple frequency table of `mweightgr` (`tab1 mweightgr`).

8-8. Include a new variable `mweightgr` in `metricauto.dta` by including the relevant commands in the do-file (`gen_metricauto.do`). Run the do-file again.

9 Commands affecting data structure

Whereas chapter 8 was concerned with single variables, this chapter describes how to modify the structure of your data. Beginners should read sections 9.1–9.4 but might want to skip some of the more complex material later in this chapter.

9.1 Safeguarding your data

When you use commands that modify your data, they affect the data in memory, not the data on disk. If you want to save the modifications, you need to save a file with a *new* name so as not to risk destroying information; see section 6.1.

If you modified your data, you must issue a new `use` command to retrieve the dataset as it was prior to the modification. However, `preserve` and `restore` (documented in [P] **preserve**) let you make temporary modifications and selections:

```
. preserve              Preserve a copy of the data currently in memory
. keep if sex == 1      The following analyses are for males only
      (analyses)
. restore               Reload the preserved dataset
```

9.2 Selecting observations and variables

You can read more about selecting observations and variables in [D] **drop**.

Selecting variables

You can remove variables from the data in memory by typing

```
. keep sex age-weight
```

and by typing

```
. drop sbp*
```

You can select only part of the data when you open a dataset:

```
. use sex age-weight using alpha.dta
```

Selecting observations

You can remove observations from the data in memory by typing

> `. keep if sex == 1`

or

> `. drop if sex != 1`

You can restrict the data in memory to the first 100 observations by typing

> `. keep in 1/100`

You can select part of the data when you open a dataset by typing

> `. use alpha.dta if sex == 1`
> `. use alpha.dta in 1/100`

Random sampling

You can keep a 10% random sample of the observations by typing

> `. sample 10`

You can keep a sample of exactly 57 observations by typing

> `. sample 57, count`

For more information, see [D] **sample**.

9.3   Renaming and reordering variables

Renaming variables

You can change the name of a variable by typing

> `. rename gender sex`

The variable name gender is changed to sex. Contents and labels are unchanged. You can read more in [D] **rename**.

Reordering variables

To change the sequence of variables in the dataset, use the following command:

> `. order id age-weight`

The new sequence of variables will be as defined, and any variables not mentioned will follow after the variables mentioned. To order the variables alphabetically, use the command

```
. aorder
```

For more information, see [D] **order**.

9.4 Sorting data

To sort your data according to mpg (primary key) and weight (secondary key), type

```
. sort mpg weight
```

sort sorts only in ascending order; gsort is more flexible but is slower. To sort by mpg (ascending) and weight (descending), type

```
. gsort mpg -weight
```

The by *varlist*: prefix and some commands like merge (see section 9.5) require sorted data. You might be confident that your data are in the right sequence and yet get the error message

```
not sorted
```

The problem is that Stata does not "know" that the sequence is right; the solution is to sort the data.

For more information about sorting, see [D] **sort** and [D] **gsort**.

9.5 Combining files

Appending files

Imagine that instead of auto.dta, you have two datasets, domestic.dta with data on 52 domestic makes, and foreign.dta with data on 22 foreign makes; you want to combine them to combined.dta (74 observations). The two datasets have the same variables; it might help to visualize the process:

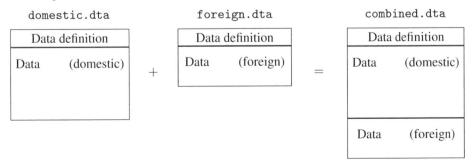

The two files have the same variables; it is only the data that differ. Combine the two files using a do-file:

```
―――――――――― gen_combined.do ――――――――――
* gen_combined.do
cd C:\docs\proj1
use domestic.dta, clear
append using foreign.dta
save combined.dta
```

Here, the dataset in memory before the `append` command was `domestic.dta`; this is called the *master* file or primary file. Labels from the secondary file (`foreign.dta`) will not replace labels in the master file, but if the master file has variables without labels, any labels from the secondary file will be copied—unless you specify the option `nolabel`.

See [D] **append** for more about combining files.

Merging files

You might have information about individuals or other study subjects from several sources; if the data from each source are in a separate file, you might want to combine them. The situation can be depicted like this:

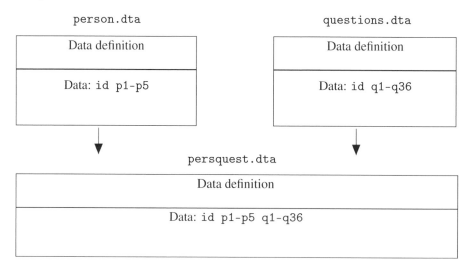

You have `person.dta` with the variables p1–p5 containing basic characteristics of the individuals, and `questions.dta` containing responses from a questionnaire in the variables q1–q36. In both datasets, the variable id uniquely identifies the individuals.

```
───────────────────────── gen_persquest.do ──────────────────
* gen_persquest.do

cd C:\docs\proj1
use person.dta, clear
merge id using questions.dta, sort

save persquest.dta
```

The files must be sorted by the matching key (id in the example) before merging; you can accomplish this task by using the `sort` option. The matching key must have the same name in both datasets, but the other variable names are typically different.

Stata creates the variable `_merge`, which takes the value 1 if its values come only from dataset 1 (the master dataset, `filea`), 2 if only dataset 2 (the using dataset, `fileb`) contributes, and 3 if both sets contribute. If you expect a 1:1 match, check for mismatches by typing

```
. tab1 _merge
. list id _merge if _merge < 3
```

The `sort` option requires that the matching key be unique in both datasets, i.e., that there be no duplicate matching keys. If there are—and if that is not an error—do not use merge's `sort` option, but use the `sort` *command* to sort both files by the matching key before merging.

In the following example, the matching key is not unique; there are duplicates. Numbers represent the matching key, and A and B represent the other variables in the input files; missing information in the result file is shown by a period:

filea	fileb	fileab	_merge
1 A	1 B	1 A B	3
2 A		2 A .	1
	3 B	3 . B	2
4 A	4 B	4 A B	3
4 A		4 A B	3
5 A	5 B	5 A B	3
	5 B	5 A B	3

For id 4, there were two observations in the master file (`filea`) but only one in `fileb`, resulting in two observations with the information from `fileb` assigned to both of them. This method enables you to distribute information about patients to each of their admissions— if that is what you desire. But what if the duplicate id 4 was an error? To check for duplicate keys before merging, sort and compare with the previous observation:

```
. sort id
. list id if id==id[_n-1]
```

Another way to check for and list observations with duplicate ID's is

```
. duplicates report id
. duplicates list id
```

merge is a lot more flexible than described here. Among other things, you can use the using file to update the information in the master file; see [D] **merge**.

9.6   Reshaping data

contract, expand

contract *varlist* creates a dataset with an observation for each combination of values in *varlist*; the variable _freq indicates the frequency of each combination; see [D] **contract**. metricauto.dta (created in exercise 8.8) includes the categorical variables foreign and mweightgr; create a contracted dataset by typing

```
. cd C:\docs\ishr
. use metricauto.dta
. contract mweightgr foreign
```

The contracted dataset has 7 observations, one for each combination of foreign and mweightgr; the variable _freq is the number of observations for that combination:

```
. list, nolabel abbrev(10)
```

	foreign	mweightgr	_freq
1.	0	1	5
2.	1	1	12
3.	0	2	18
4.	1	2	9
5.	0	3	27
6.	1	3	1
7.	0	4	2

This is a tabular form of the data; you will want use frequency weighting when analyzing data like the following:

```
. tab2 mweightgr foreign [fweight=_freq]
-> tabulation of mweightgr by foreign
    Weight (kg) │      Car type
        grouped │ 0. Domest  1. Foreig │    Total
────────────────┼──────────────────────┼──────────
    1. -999 kg  │      5          12   │      17
 2. 1000-1499 kg│     18           9   │      27
 3. 1500-1999 kg│     27           1   │      28
    4. 2000 kg+ │      2           0   │       2
────────────────┼──────────────────────┼──────────
          Total │     52          22   │      74
```

With expand (see [D] **expand**) you can create the opposite effect; typing

```
. expand _freq
```

creates a dataset with 74 observations that can be analyzed without weighting.

Look at the example from section 4.5 about weighting observations. You have access to tabular information of the following type:

	Cases	Controls
Exposed	21	30
Unexposed	23	100
Total	44	130

You can create the corresponding contracted dataset by using the input command (see section 6.2)

```
. input expos case pop
  1 1 21
  1 0 30
  0 1 23
  0 0 100
  end
```

and analyze by typing (see section 10.3)

```
. tab2 expos case [fweight=pop], chi2
```

You can obtain the same result by expanding the 4 observations to 174 observations:

```
. expand pop
. tab2 expos case, chi2
```

collapse

The collapse command (see [D] **collapse**) is similar to contract: you can use it to create an aggregated dataset, not with the characteristics of each individual but of groups of individuals.

Imagine, for example, that you have data on the members of various trade unions. You now want to create a file characterizing each union by the proportion of males and by the mean age and median income among members. sex is coded 0 for females, 1 for males:

```
. collapse (mean) meanage=age pmale=sex (median) medinc=income,
> by(union)
```

The aggregated dataset has one observation for each union, with the mean age, the proportion males (the mean of a 0/1-coded variable is the proportion of 1s), and the median income.

A collapsed file like this one can again be merged with the original data to compare members with general characteristics of their union. More simply, we could obtain the same results by typing (see section 8.3)

```
. sort union
. by union: egen pmale = mean(sex)
. by union: egen meanage = mean(age)
. by union: egen medinc = median(income)
```

reshape

With repeated measurements and paired observations (not to mention dentistry, where a person may have 32 teeth) some analyses require a "wide" and some a "long" data structure. In anklebp1.dta (to be used in chapter 15), the data structure is wide; one observation includes two blood pressure measurements at each site:

```
. cd C:\docs\ishr
. use anklebp1.dta
(Ankle blood pressure data)
. list in 1/3
```

	id	adp1	adp2	atp1	atp2
1.	1	105	110	105	105
2.	2	110	110	110	110
3.	4	140	130	150	160

For reasons explained in section 15.1, we need a long structure with one observation for each measurement:

```
. reshape long adp atp, i(id) j(meas)
(note: j = 1 2)
```

Data	wide	->	long
Number of obs.	107	->	214
Number of variables	5	->	4
j variable (2 values)		->	meas
xij variables:			
	adp1 adp2	->	adp
	atp1 atp2	->	atp

The dataset now has the desired long structure with one observation per measurement:

```
. list in 1/6, sepby(id)
```

	id	meas	adp	atp
1.	1	1	105	105
2.	1	2	110	105
3.	2	1	110	110
4.	2	2	110	110
5.	4	1	140	150
6.	4	2	130	160

We could do the opposite by typing

```
. reshape wide adp atp, i(id) j(meas)
```

For more information, see [D] **reshape**. Also see a discussion of long and wide data structures in section 11.2 and an example of reshaping data in section 15.1.

xpose

You can transpose observations and variables, changing observations to variables and variables to observations. This ability may be useful for restructuring data such as for use in a graph:

```
. xpose, clear
```

`clear` is mandatory to remind you that this command destroys your original data in memory. Read more in [D] **xpose**.

10 Description and simple analysis

10.1 Overview of a dataset

The lbw dataset

For most analyses in this chapter, we will use the dataset `lbw.dta` from Hosmer and Lemeshow (2000) about predictors of low birthweight. The study was designed with an excess of children with low birthweight, but we will ignore that in this chapter. The dataset is used for several examples in the Stata reference manuals; you can obtain such datasets from the Internet by typing, for example,

```
. webuse lbw.dta
```

In this dataset, a common convention was used for yes–no variables, coding No as 0 and Yes as 1; no value labels were defined for this rather obvious coding. I chose, however, to add value labels to these variables and save the dataset in C:\docs\ishr as `lbw1.dta`. Generally, you should make such modifications to the dataset using a do-file:

```
────────────────── gen_lbw1.do ──────────────────
* gen_lbw1.do adds labels to lbw.dta and saves lbw1.dta

webuse lbw.dta, clear

* Add value label yesno to the appropriate variables
label define yesno  0 No  1 Yes
label values low yesno
label values smoke yesno
label values ht yesno
label values ui yesno
numlabel _all, add                      // include code in value labels

* compress and save
compress
cd C:\docs\ishr
save lbw1.dta, replace
```

describe

describe (see [D] **describe**) gives you information about how variables are defined in a dataset: the number of observations and variables, the file size in bytes, variable names, storage types (see section 5.4), display formats (see section 5.2), variable and value labels (see section 7.1), and the sorting status of the dataset. This dataset was not sorted:

```
. cd C:\docs\ishr

. use lbw1.dta, clear
(Hosmer & Lemeshow data)

. describe

Contains data from lbw1.dta
  obs:           189                          Hosmer & Lemeshow data
 vars:            11                          2 Apr 2005 21:10
 size:         3,402 (99.9% of memory free)

              storage   display    value
variable name   type    format     label     variable label

id              int     %8.0g                 identification code
low             byte    %8.0g      yesno      birthweight<2500g
age             byte    %8.0g                 age of mother
lwt             int     %8.0g                 weight at last menstrual period
race            byte    %8.0g      race       race
smoke           byte    %8.0g      yesno      smoked during pregnancy
ptl             byte    %8.0g                 premature labor history (count)
ht              byte    %8.0g      yesno      has history of hypertension
ui              byte    %8.0g      yesno      presence, uterine irritability
ftv             byte    %8.0g                 number of visits to physician
                                                during 1st trimester
bwt             int     %8.0g                 birthweight (grams)

Sorted by:
```

Use label list to see the value labels (the double numbers are due to numlabel, which added the code to the value label):

```
. label list
yesno:
           0 0. No
           1 1. Yes
race:
           1 1. white
           2 2. black
           3 3. other
```

codebook

codebook (see [D] **codebook**) gives you more detailed information about each variable. If you do not specify a variable list, Stata displays information for all variables, and the output may be a bit overwhelming. Here we ask for a single variable:

```
. codebook bwt
```

bwt	birthweight (grams)

```
              type:  numeric (int)

             range:  [709,4990]              units:  1
     unique values:  133               missing .:  0/189

              mean:  2944.29
         std. dev:  729.016

       percentiles:       10%      25%      50%      75%      90%
                         1970     2414     2977     3475     3884
```

The compact option is useful for obtaining an overview of the dataset. For each variable this command displays the number of nonmissing observations, the number of unique values, and the minimum and maximum values:

```
. codebook, compact
Variable    Obs Unique      Mean  Min   Max  Label

id          189    189  121.0794    4   226  identification code
low         189      2  .3121693    0     1  birthweight<2500g
age         189     24   23.2381   14    45  age of mother
lwt         189     76  129.8201   80   250  weight at last menstrual period
race        189      3  1.846561    1     3  race
smoke       189      2  .3915344    0     1  smoked during pregnancy
ptl         189      4  .1957672    0     3  premature labor history (count)
ht          189      2  .0634921    0     1  has history of hypertension
ui          189      2  .1481481    0     1  presence, uterine irritability
ftv         189      6  .7936508    0     6  number of visits to physician du...
bwt         189    133  2944.286  709  4990  birthweight (grams)
```

summarize

summarize is another command that is useful for an initial overview of the data; see [R] **summarize**.

(*Continued on next page*)

```
. use lbw1.dta, clear
(Hosmer & Lemeshow data)

. summarize
    Variable |        Obs        Mean    Std. Dev.       Min        Max
-------------+-------------------------------------------------------
          id |        189    121.0794    63.30363          4        226
         low |        189    .3121693    .4646093          0          1
         age |        189     23.2381    5.298678         14         45
         lwt |        189    129.8201    30.57515         80        250
        race |        189    1.846561    .9183422          1          3
-------------+-------------------------------------------------------
       smoke |        189    .3915344    .4893898          0          1
         ptl |        189    .1957672    .4933419          0          3
          ht |        189    .0634921    .2444936          0          1
          ui |        189    .1481481    .3561903          0          1
         ftv |        189    .7936508    1.059286          0          6
-------------+-------------------------------------------------------
         bwt |        189    2944.286     729.016        709       4990
```

Most often, I prefer `codebook, compact` to `summarize` because it also displays the variable labels.

10.2 Listing observations

list

Listing observations is useful to help you examine data, check the result of calculations, and locate errors. Read more in [D] **list**. The following lists all variables in all observations:

```
. use lbw1.dta, clear
(Hosmer & Lemeshow data)

. list
```

	id	low	age	lwt	race	smoke	ptl	ht	ui	ftv	bwt
1.	85	0. No	19	182	2. black	0. No	0	0. No	1. Yes	0	2523
2.	86	0. No	33	155	3. other	0. No	0	0. No	0. No	3	2551
3.	87	0. No	20	105	1. white	1. Yes	0	0. No	0. No	1	2557
4.	88	0. No	21	108	1. white	1. Yes	0	0. No	1. Yes	2	2594
5.	89	0. No	18	107	1. white	1. Yes	0	0. No	1. Yes	0	2600
6.	91	0. No	21	124	3. other	0. No	0	0. No	0. No	0	2622

(output omitted)

Often listing the value labels creates more noise than clarity. To list the codes rather than the labels, restricting to the variables `id`-`smoke` in the first 5 observations, type

```
. list id-smoke in 1/5, nolabel
```

	id	low	age	lwt	race	smoke
1.	85	0	19	182	2	0
2.	86	0	33	155	3	0
3.	87	0	20	105	1	1
4.	88	0	21	108	1	1
5.	89	0	18	107	1	1

By default, list draws a separator line for each 5 observations. You can change this setting by using the separator() option. separator(0) drops separator lines; separator(10) draws a line for each 10 observations. The sepby(*varlist*) option draws a separator line each time the values in *varlist* change. The mean, sum, and N options (capital N) display a bottom line with the requested statistic. N displays the number of nonmissing values for each variable. If you supply a *varlist*, as in mean(bwt), the statistic will only apply to these variables:

```
. sort race smoke
. list race smoke bwt if bwt<1800, sepby(race) N mean(bwt)
```

	race	smoke	bwt
22.	1. white	0. No	1021
81.	1. white	1. Yes	1790
104.	2. black	0. No	1701
122.	2. black	1. Yes	1135
139.	3. other	0. No	1330
141.	3. other	0. No	1588
142.	3. other	0. No	1729
145.	3. other	0. No	1474
152.	3. other	0. No	1588
185.	3. other	1. Yes	709
Mean			1406.5
N	10	10	10

You can get rid of the lines by using the clean option and drop observation numbers using the noobs option:

```
. list id-smoke in 1/5, nolabel clean noobs
    id   low   age   lwt   race   smoke
    85    0    19    182     2      0
    86    0    33    155     3      0
    87    0    20    105     1      1
    88    0    21    108     1      1
    89    0    18    107     1      1
```

When you need to list more variables than can fit on a line, the list output becomes less useful:

```
. sysuse auto.dta, clear
(1978 Automobile Data)
. list in 1/2, nolabel
```

1.	make	price	mpg	rep78	headroom	trunk	weight	length
	AMC Concord	4,099	22	3	2.5	11	2,930	186

	turn	displa~t	gear_r~o	foreign
	40	121	3.58	0

2.	make	price	mpg	rep78	headroom	trunk	weight	length
	AMC Pacer	4,749	17	3	3.0	11	3,350	173

	turn	displa~t	gear_r~o	foreign
	40	258	2.53	0

Here you may find a user-generated facility, `slist`, to be convenient; you can find and install it by typing

```
. findit slist
```

If the variables do not fit on one line, `slist` splits the variables into blocks that do. In the following command, the `id(make)` option lets the identifying variable `make` occur in each block. The `decimal(2)` option lets floating-point numbers be displayed with two decimals. `nolabel` is the default; you can use the `label` option to display labels rather than codes.

```
. slist in 1/2, id(make) decimal(2)
         make            price  mpg  rep78  headroom  trunk  weight  length  turn
   1. AMC Concord         4099   22      3      2.50     11    2930     186    40
   2. AMC Pacer           4749   17      3      3.00     11    3350     173    40

         make         displacement  gear_ratio  foreign
   1. AMC Concord              121        3.58        0
   2. AMC Pacer                258        2.53        0
```

browse

The `browse` command lets you see observations and variables in the Data window, much like the `list` command, but `browse` is not good for printing the results:

```
. browse id-smoke in 1/5
```

In the Data window, string variables are displayed in red and value labels in blue. Right-clicking in the Data window lets you toggle between display of codes and value labels.

10.3   Simple tables for categorical variables

`tab1` for one-way tables (frequency tables) and `tab2` for two-way contingency tables (cross tables) are both variations of the `tabulate` command (`tabulate` with one variable creates a frequency table like `tab1`; `tabulate` with two variables creates a cross table like `tab2`).

tab1

tab1 (see [R] **tabulate oneway**) creates one-way tables (frequency tables) like the following:

```
. cd C:\docs\ishr

. use lbw1.dta
(Hosmer & Lemeshow data)

. tab1 race

-> tabulation of race
```

race	Freq.	Percent	Cum.
1. white	96	50.79	50.79
2. black	26	13.76	64.55
3. other	67	35.45	100.00
Total	189	100.00	

tab1 allows you to specify several tables in the *varlist*, e.g.:

```
. tab1 low race-ftv
```

But beware that if you try to tabulate variables with many values (like id and bwt), you get huge but most often useless tables.

tab1 calculates no statistics. Two often used options are

- nolabel to display codes rather than value labels.
- missing to include tabulation of missing values. The default is to omit them.

proportion

proportion (see [R] **proportion**) estimates proportions with confidence intervals:

```
. use lbw1.dta
(Hosmer & Lemeshow data)

. proportion race
```

```
Proportion estimation              Number of obs   =     189

        _prop_1: race = 1. white
        _prop_2: race = 2. black
        _prop_3: race = 3. other
```

	Proportion	Std. Err.	Binomial Wald [95% Conf. Interval]	
race				
_prop_1	.5079365	.0364617	.43601	.5798631
_prop_2	.1375661	.0251212	.0880106	.1871217
_prop_3	.3544974	.034888	.285675	.4233197

With the over() option you can study subgroups; here you can see the estimated proportions of smokers and nonsmokers by race:

```
. proportion smoke, over(race)
Proportion estimation                    Number of obs    =      189
        _prop_1: smoke = 0. No
        _prop_2: smoke = 1. Yes

      _subpop_1: race = 1. white
      _subpop_2: race = 2. black
      _subpop_3: race = 3. other
```

	Proportion	Std. Err.	Binomial Wald [95% Conf. Interval]	
Over	Proportion	Std. Err.	[95% Conf.	Interval]
_prop_1				
_subpop_1	.4583333	.0511205	.3574899	.5591768
_subpop_2	.6153846	.0973009	.4234429	.8073264
_subpop_3	.8208955	.0471982	.7277894	.9140016
_prop_2				
_subpop_1	.5416667	.0511205	.4408232	.6425101
_subpop_2	.3846154	.0973009	.1926736	.5765571
_subpop_3	.1791045	.0471982	.0859984	.2722106

tab2

tab2 (see [R] **tabulate twoway**) creates two-way contingency tables (cross tables):

```
. use lbw1.dta, clear
(Hosmer & Lemeshow data)

. tab2 low race, column chi2 exact

-> tabulation of low by race
```

Key
frequency
column percentage

birthweigh t<2500g	race 1. white	2. black	3. other	Total
0. No	73	15	42	130
	76.04	57.69	62.69	68.78
1. Yes	23	11	25	59
	23.96	42.31	37.31	31.22
Total	96	26	67	189
	100.00	100.00	100.00	100.00

```
          Pearson chi2(2) =   5.0048   Pr = 0.082
          Fisher's exact =              0.079
```

Some frequently used options are

- column (or col) displays column percent.
- row displays row percent.
- chi2 calculates Pearson's chi-squared test.
- exact calculates Fisher's exact test.
- nolabel displays codes rather than value labels.
- missing includes tabulation of missing values. The default is to omit them.

You can request a three-way table (a two-way table for each value of smoke) by typing

```
. by smoke, sort: tab2 low race
```

```
-> smoke = 0. No
-> tabulation of low by race
```

birthweigh t<2500g	1. white	race 2. black	3. other	Total
0. No	40	11	35	86
1. Yes	4	5	20	29
Total	44	16	55	115

```
-> smoke = 1. Yes
-> tabulation of low by race
```

birthweigh t<2500g	1. white	race 2. black	3. other	Total
0. No	33	4	7	44
1. Yes	19	6	5	30
Total	52	10	12	74

tab2 allows you to have many variables in the *varlist*; the command

```
. tab2 smoke low race
```

gives you three two-way tables, one for each possible combination of two variables. But be careful, as you can easily produce a huge number of tables. Imagine that you want 10 tables, each of the variables q1-q10 by treatment. With tabulate, you must issue 10 commands to obtain the desired result. If you call tab2 with 11 variables, you get 55 tables—all possible pairs of the 11 variables.

The foreach command (see section 17.4) lets you circumvent the problem:

```
. foreach Q of varlist q1-q10 {
  tab2 'Q' treat
  }
```

The local macro Q is a stand-in for q1 to q10, and the construct generates 10 commands:

```
. tab2 q1 treat
. tab2 q2 treat
. ...
```

table

table is a flexible tool that allows you to build complex tables, but it calculates no statistics; see [R] **table**. Here is the same three-way contingency table that we obtained above:

```
. use lbw1.dta, clear
(Hosmer & Lemeshow data)
. table low race smoke
```

birthweig ht<2500g	smoked during pregnancy and race					
	0. No			1. Yes		
	1. white	2. black	3. other	1. white	2. black	3. other
0. No	40	11	35	33	4	7
1. Yes	4	5	20	19	6	5

table has several options, giving you control over the format of tables. Here the by() option organizes the tables for smokers and nonsmokers vertically, row and col add totals, and stubwidth() determines the width of the stub:

```
. table low race, by(smoke) row col stubwidth(20)
```

smoked during pregnancy and birthweight<2500g	race			
	1. white	2. black	3. other	Total
0. No				
0. No	40	11	35	86
1. Yes	4	5	20	29
Total	44	16	55	115
1. Yes				
0. No	33	4	7	44
1. Yes	19	6	5	30
Total	52	10	12	74

Section 10.4 shows you how to use table for continuous variables.

tabm

tabm is a user-written command that is useful for compact tabulation of several similar categorical variables. It is part of the tab_chi package; you can find and install it by typing

```
. findit tabm
```

In rvary2.dta, five different raters could rate 10 objects with characters from 1 to 3:

```
. webuse rvary2.dta
. tabm rater*
```

		Values		
Variable	1	2	3	Total
rater1	8	1	1	10
rater2	5	3	2	10
rater3	4	3	2	9
rater4	2	2	4	8
rater5	1	2	7	10
Total	20	11	16	47

groups

groups lets you tabulate combinations of several categorical variables. It is a user-written command (Cox 2003b), so you must first install it from the SSC archives (see section 2.2):

```
. ssc install groups
```

Having done that, you can specify the variables to be included:

```
. use lbw1.dta, clear
(Hosmer & Lemeshow data)
. groups low race smoke
```

low	race	smoke	Freq.	Percent
0. No	1. white	0. No	40	21.16
0. No	1. white	1. Yes	33	17.46
0. No	2. black	0. No	11	5.82
0. No	2. black	1. Yes	4	2.12
0. No	3. other	0. No	35	18.52
0. No	3. other	1. Yes	7	3.70
1. Yes	1. white	0. No	4	2.12
1. Yes	1. white	1. Yes	19	10.05
1. Yes	2. black	0. No	5	2.65
1. Yes	2. black	1. Yes	6	3.17
1. Yes	3. other	0. No	20	10.58
1. Yes	3. other	1. Yes	5	2.65

groups is a hybrid of a list and a table, and many list options apply, such as sum, sepby(), and nolabel. A particularly useful option is show(); the arguments can be frequency (f), percent (p), cumulative frequency (F) and percent (P), and reverse cumulative frequency (RF) and percent (RP):

```
. groups low smoke, nolabel sum sepby(low) show(f p F P RF RP)
```

low	smoke	Freq.	Percent	# <=	% <=	# >	% >
0	0	86	45.50	86	45.50	103	54.50
0	1	44	23.28	130	68.78	59	31.22
1	0	29	15.34	159	84.13	30	15.87
1	1	30	15.87	189	100.00	0	0.00
Sum		189	100.00				

10.4   Analyzing continuous variables

Description of distributions

For the lbw1.dta dataset, the summarize output (section 10.1) displayed the mean birthweight (bwt) = 2,944 g and SD = 729 g. The detail option gives more information about percentiles, etc. The median (50% percentile) is 2,977 g; the four smallest and the four largest observations are displayed, too:

```
. use lbw1.dta, clear
(Hosmer & Lemeshow data)

. summarize bwt, detail

                          birthweight (grams)
```

	Percentiles	Smallest		
1%	1021	709		
5%	1790	1021		
10%	1970	1135	Obs	189
25%	2414	1330	Sum of Wgt.	189
50%	2977		Mean	2944.286
		Largest	Std. Dev.	729.016
75%	3475	4174		
90%	3884	4238	Variance	531464.4
95%	3997	4593	Skewness	-.2069782
99%	4593	4990	Kurtosis	2.888821

Figure 10.1 is a histogram with the corresponding normal curve (see [R] **histogram**). We made a few extra modifications with this graph (see gph_fig10_1.do, available at this book's web site), but the main command is

```
. histogram bwt, frequency normal
```

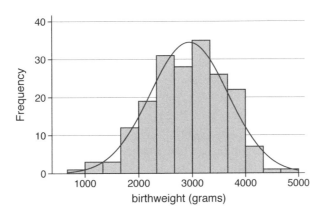

Figure 10.1: Histogram with normal curve

The birthweight distribution does not seem far from a normal distribution. Some people prefer (I do not) to assess agreement with a normal distribution by a so-called Q–Q plot (see [R] **diagnostic plots**); the main command for that is

```
. qnorm bwt
```

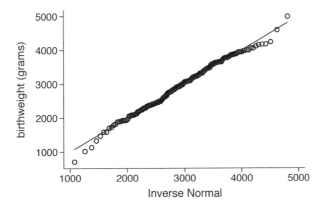

Figure 10.2: Q–Q plot

The conclusion drawn from the Q–Q plot would be the same as that from the histogram, with only minor departures from a normal distribution.

There are also formal tests for departure from a normal distribution, such as the Shapiro–Wilk test (see [R] **swilk**):

```
. swilk bwt
```

	Shapiro-Wilk W test for normal data				
Variable	Obs	W	V	z	Prob>z
bwt	189	0.99263	1.047	0.106	0.45774

The departure from a normal distribution was not at all statistically significant (Pr = 0.46). Significance testing for normality may, however, be misleading: With large datasets, even unimportant departures from normality become statistically significant, and the most important tool is visual inspection.

Continuous distributions are often displayed by box-and-whisker plots (see [G] **graph box**). The box displays the interquartile range (the 25th and 75th percentile) and the median. The whiskers display the upper and lower values within 1.5 times the interquartile range beyond the 25th and 75th percentile. Any outliers beyond those limits get their own markers. The main command for the box plot shown in figure 10.3 is

```
. graph box bwt, over(smoke)
```

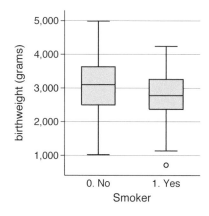

Figure 10.3: Box-and-whisker plot

Transformations

Some analyses, such as *t* tests and linear regression, require the dependent variable to have a normal distribution (conditional on the values of the independent variables), and a transformation may be required to obtain that. gladder (see [R] **ladder**) displays various transformations; the name refers to the "ladder of powers" (Tukey 1977):

```
. sysuse auto.dta, clear
(1978 Automobile Data)
. gladder mpg, frequency
```

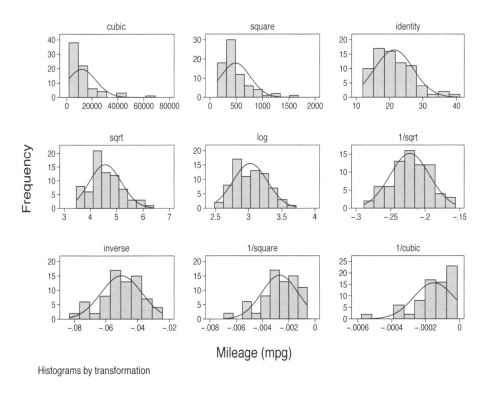

Histograms by transformation

Figure 10.4: `gladder` displays the effect of various transformations.

You can obtain a statistical test of normality for the transformations by using `ladder`:

```
. ladder mpg
```

Transformation	formula	chi2(2)	P(chi2)
cubic	mpg^3	43.59	0.000
square	mpg^2	27.03	0.000
raw	mpg	10.95	0.004
square-root	sqrt(mpg)	4.94	0.084
log	log(mpg)	0.87	0.647
reciprocal root	1/sqrt(mpg)	0.20	0.905
reciprocal	1/mpg	2.36	0.307
reciprocal square	1/(mpg^2)	11.99	0.002
reciprocal cubic	1/(mpg^3)	24.30	0.000

Now you could decide to choose the transformation with the least-significant departure from normality (1/sqrt(mpg)), but you might have a problem in interpreting and communicating it. The inverse (1/mpg) is a better choice because it has a direct interpretation: gas consumption in gallons per mile.

With large datasets, even small and unimportant departures may become significant. Look at the graphs, not the *p*-values, and consider the interpretability of a transformation.

mean

mean (see [R] **mean**) estimates means. With the over() option, mean displays the mean for subgroups:

```
. cd C:\docs\ishr
. use lbw1.dta, clear
(Hosmer & Lemeshow data)
. mean bwt, over(smoke race)

Mean estimation                    Number of obs    =      189

          Over: smoke race
     _subpop_1: 0. No 1. white
     _subpop_2: 0. No 2. black
     _subpop_3: 0. No 3. other
     _subpop_4: 1. Yes 1. white
     _subpop_5: 1. Yes 2. black
     _subpop_6: 1. Yes 3. other
```

Over	Mean	Std. Err.	[95% Conf. Interval]	
bwt				
_subpop_1	3428.75	107.0514	3217.574	3639.926
_subpop_2	2854.5	155.3136	2548.119	3160.881
_subpop_3	2814.236	95.50185	2625.843	3002.629
_subpop_4	2827.385	86.90549	2655.949	2998.82
_subpop_5	2504	201.455	2106.597	2901.403
_subpop_6	2757.167	233.8397	2295.88	3218.454

tabstat

tabstat (see [R] **tabstat**) displays summary statistics for numeric variables, typically broken down by another variable; you can consider it an extended summarize. In its simplest form, it displays only means:

```
. use lbw1.dta, clear
(Hosmer & Lemeshow data)
. tabstat age lwt bwt, by(race)

Summary statistics: mean
  by categories of: race (race)
```

race	age	lwt	bwt
1. white	24.29167	132.0521	3103.01
2. black	21.53846	146.8077	2719.692
3. other	22.38806	120.0299	2804.015
Total	23.2381	129.8201	2944.286

`tabstat` offers several summary statistics:

Statistic	Definition	Statistic	Definition
`mean`	Mean	`cv`	Coefficient of variation (`sd`/`mean`)
`n`	Number of nonmissing observations	`semean`	Standard error of mean
`sum`	Sum	`skew`	Skewness
`min`	Minimum	`kurt`	Kurtosis
`max`	Maximum	`p1`	1st percentile
`range`	Range (`max-min`)	`p5 p10`	`p25 p50 p75 p90 p95 p99`
`sd`	Standard deviation	`iqr`	Interquartile range (`p75-p25`)
`var`	Variance	`q`	Quartiles (`p25 p50 p75`)

To display n, mean, sd, cv, semean, and median (or p50) for three variables, type

```
. tabstat age lwt bwt, by(smoke) stat(n mean sd cv semean median)
> longstub

    smoke      stats |       age       lwt       bwt
    -----------------+------------------------------
    0. No        N   |       115       115       115
              mean   |  23.42609  130.9043  3054.957
                sd   |  5.467706  28.41916   752.409
                cv   | .2334024  .2170987  .2462912
           se(mean)  | .5098662    2.6501   70.1625
               p50   |        23       124      3100
    -----------------+------------------------------
    1. Yes       N   |        74        74        74
              mean   |  22.94595  128.1351  2772.297
                sd   |  5.047424  33.78673  659.8075
                cv   | .2199702  .2636805  .2380003
           se(mean)  | .5867511  3.927628  76.70106
               p50   |        22       120    2775.5
    -----------------+------------------------------
    Total        N   |       189       189       189
              mean   |   23.2381  129.8201  2944.286
                sd   |  5.298678  30.57515   729.016
                cv   | .2280169  .2355194  .2476037
           se(mean)  | .3854221  2.224015  53.02811
               p50   |        23       121      2977
    -----------------+------------------------------
```

The `longstub` option shows the name of the statistics in the stub.

You can display the statistics columnwise by using the `col(stat)` option. And you can control the display format by using the `format()` option:

```
. tabstat age lwt bwt, stat(n mean sd q) col(stat) format(%8.2f)
    variable |        N       mean         sd        p25        p50        p75
-------------+------------------------------------------------------------------
         age |   189.00      23.24       5.30      19.00      23.00      26.00
         lwt |   189.00     129.82      30.58     110.00     121.00     140.00
         bwt |   189.00    2944.29     729.02    2414.00    2977.00    3475.00
```

tabulate, summarize()

tabulate with the summarize() option (see [R] **tabulate, summarize**) is similar to tabstat, but it is less flexible; the following command displays a table identical to the table produced by oneway with the tabulate option (see *oneway* later in this section):

. tabulate race, summarize(bwt)

You can also display the distribution of a continuous variable by two categorical variables:

. tabulate race smoke, summarize(bwt)

```
    Means, Standard Deviations and Frequencies of birthweight (grams)

             | smoked during
             |   pregnancy
       race  |   0. No    1. Yes |     Total
-------------+-------------------+-----------
   1. white  | 3428.75  2827.3846| 3103.0104
             |710.09892 626.68443|727.87244
             |      44         52|        96
-------------+-------------------+-----------
   2. black  |  2854.5       2504| 2719.6923
             |621.25432 637.05677|638.68388
             |      16         10|        26
-------------+-------------------+-----------
   3. other  |2814.2364  2757.1667| 2804.0149
             |708.2607  810.04465|721.30115
             |      55         12|        67
-------------+-------------------+-----------
       Total |3054.9565  2772.2973| 2944.2857
             |752.40901 659.80748|729.01602
             |     115         74|       189
```

table

You can use table (see [R] **table**) to build complex tables. In section 10.3, I showed three-way contingency tables; here I only show a simple example of comparing means between subgroups:

```
. table race smoke, contents(mean bwt) format(%9.1f)
```

race	smoked during pregnancy	
	0. No	1. Yes
1. white	3428.8	2827.4
2. black	2854.5	2504.0
3. other	2814.2	2757.2

As you see, there are several partly overlapping possibilities to tabulate means, etc. My favorite is tabstat, which is the most flexible.

oneway

oneway compares means between two or more groups (analysis of variance); see [R] **oneway**.

```
. oneway bwt race, tabulate
```

race	Summary of birthweight (grams)		
	Mean	Std. Dev.	Freq.
1. white	3103.0104	727.87244	96
2. black	2719.6923	638.68388	26
3. other	2804.0149	721.30115	67
Total	2944.2857	729.01602	189

	Analysis of Variance				
Source	SS	df	MS	F	Prob > F
Between groups	5048361.06	2	2524180.53	4.95	0.0081
Within groups	94866937.5	186	510037.298		
Total	99915298.6	188	531464.354		

```
Bartlett's test for equal variances:  chi2(2) =   0.6560  Prob>chi2 = 0.720
```

The descriptive table displays the birthweight distribution (mean and SD) for each race. The ANOVA table tests and rejects (Pr = 0.008) the null hypothesis that there is no difference between means. Among the options are tabulate, which displays a descriptive table, as above, and noanova, which suppresses display of the ANOVA table.

For more complex ANOVAs, see [R] **anova**.

ttest

The family of t test commands allow you to compare the means of a normally distributed variable between two groups or to make a paired comparison of two variables; see [R] **ttest**:

. `ttest bmi, by(sex)`	Comparison of two groups; equal variances assumed
. `ttest bmi, by(sex) unequal`	Unequal variances (see `sdtest`)
. `ttest prebmi==postbmi`	Paired comparison of two variables
. `ttest bmidiff==0`	One-sample t test

To compare mean birthweights for children born to smoking and nonsmoking mothers:

```
. use lbw1.dta, clear
(Hosmer & Lemeshow data)

. ttest bwt, by(smoke)
```

Two-sample t test with equal variances

Group	Obs	Mean	Std. Err.	Std. Dev.	[95% Conf. Interval]	
0. No	115	3054.957	70.1625	752.409	2915.965	3193.948
1. Yes	74	2772.297	76.70106	659.8075	2619.432	2925.162
combined	189	2944.286	53.02811	729.016	2839.679	3048.892
diff		282.6592	106.9544		71.66693	493.6515

```
    diff = mean(0. No) - mean(1. Yes)                        t =   2.6428
Ho: diff = 0                                degrees of freedom =      187

    Ha: diff < 0                 Ha: diff != 0                 Ha: diff > 0
 Pr(T < t) = 0.9955         Pr(|T| > |t|) = 0.0089         Pr(T > t) = 0.0045
```

The middle p-value (Pr = 0.0089) is the result of a two-sided test; the smaller of the two others (Pr = 0.0045) is the one-sided result.

In [R] **ttest** the headings for paired and two-sample tests are less than helpful, the paired t test being explained under the heading *Two-sample mean comparison test*, and the two-sample t test being under the heading *Group mean comparison test*. Otherwise, the manual's examples are good and illustrative.

sdtest

To test whether the variances (or standard deviations) can be considered equal, use `sdtest` (see [R] **sdtest**). To compare standard deviations between two groups, type

```
. sdtest bwt, by(smoke)
```
Variance ratio test

Group	Obs	Mean	Std. Err.	Std. Dev.	[95% Conf. Interval]	
0. No	115	3054.957	70.1625	752.409	2915.965	3193.948
1. Yes	74	2772.297	76.70106	659.8075	2619.432	2925.162
combined	189	2944.286	53.02811	729.016	2839.679	3048.892

```
      ratio = sd(0. No) / sd(1. Yes)                              f =    1.3004
Ho: ratio = 1                                  degrees of freedom =  114, 73

     Ha: ratio < 1              Ha: ratio != 1                 Ha: ratio > 1
   Pr(F < f) = 0.8862        2*Pr(F > f) = 0.2275           Pr(F > f) = 0.1138
```

Again, the middle p-value is the interesting two-sided test ($Pr = 0.23$), and you can consider the standard deviations to be equal and use an ordinary t test. You could have also used oneway (see above) and looked at Bartlett's test for equal variances.

You can compare the standard deviations of two variables by typing

```
. sdtest prebmi==postbmi
```

Despite the similarity with the syntax for a paired t test, sdtest makes an unpaired comparison. A test for paired comparisons, sdpair, is shown in section 15.2.

Nonparametric tests

For an overview of available tests, select

> Help ▷ Search...   and type nonparametric

and you will see, for example,

kwallis	Kruskall–Wallis equality of populations rank test
signrank	Sign, rank, and median tests (Wilcoxon, Mann–Whitney)

Another good method for searching is to use the menu system; selecting

> Statistics ▷ Summaries, tables, & tests ▷ Nonparametric tests of hypotheses

will help you find several tests. One of the options is the Mann–Whitney two-sample rank-sum test; filling in the dialog to compare birthweight among smoking and nonsmoking mothers, we get:

```
. use lbw1.dta
(Hosmer & Lemeshow data)

. ranksum bwt, by(smoke)

Two-sample Wilcoxon rank-sum (Mann-Whitney) test

        smoke |     obs   rank sum   expected
--------------+----------------------------------
        0. No |     115   11915.5      10925
        1. Yes |      74    6039.5       7030
--------------+----------------------------------
     combined |     189    17955       17955

unadjusted variance     134741.67
adjustment for ties        -11.98
                        ----------
adjusted variance       134729.69

Ho: bwt(smoke==0. No) = bwt(smoke==1. Yes)
           z =    2.699
    Prob > |z| =   0.0070
```

Nonparametric tests are based on the ranks rather than the values of the observations, and you can obtain only *p*-values, not effect estimates. Also, if the requirements for a parametric test are fulfilled, the parametric test typically will have better power than its nonparametric cousin.

10.5   Estimating confidence intervals

Many estimating commands display confidence intervals for the estimates. The default is to use 95% confidence intervals; the level() option is common to many commands and lets you choose the confidence interval, e.g., 99%:

```
. ttest bwt, by(smoke) level(99)
```

ci

ci lets you calculate confidence intervals for means, proportions, and rates; see [R] **ci**.

To estimate the mean of the continuous variable crea with a 99% confidence interval, type

```
. cd C:\docs\ishr
. use ras.dta, clear
. ci crea, level(99)

    Variable |     Obs     Mean    Std. Err.    [99% Conf. Interval]
-------------+----------------------------------------------------
        crea |     437   93.12815   1.169739    90.10185   96.15444
```

To estimate a proportion with a 95% confidence interval, use the binomial option. The variable must be coded 0/1:

```
. ci stenosis, binomial
```

Variable	Obs	Mean	Std. Err.	— Binomial Exact — [95% Conf. Interval]	
stenosis	437	.228833	.0200952	.1902529	.2711286

To estimate a confidence interval for a rate, use the `poisson` option, and state the time-at-risk variable as an argument for the `exposure()` option:

```
. use compliance2.dta, clear
. ci died, poisson exposure(risktime)
```

Variable	Exposure	Mean	Std. Err.	— Poisson Exact — [95% Conf. Interval]	
died	2634.032	.0391036	.003853	.0319176	.0474244

cii

cii is the immediate form of `ci`; see [R] **ci**. You can use the dialogs to produce the results:

```
. db cii
```

The commands have the following formats:

Normal distribution

```
. cii  N    mean    SD
. cii 372 37.58 16.51
```

Variable	Obs	Mean	Std. Err.	[95% Conf. Interval]	
	372	37.58	.8560036	35.89677	39.26323

Binomial distribution

```
. cii  N events, binomial
. cii 153 40, binomial
```

Variable	Obs	Mean	Std. Err.	— Binomial Exact — [95% Conf. Interval]	
	153	.2614379	.0355248	.1938062	.3385499

The "Mean" expresses the proportion events (40/153).

Poisson distribution

```
. cii divisor events, poisson
. cii 2471 40, poisson
```

Variable	Exposure	Mean	Std. Err.	— Poisson Exact — [95% Conf. Interval]	
	2471	.0161878	.0025595	.0115648	.0220432

The divisor ("Exposure") may be a time at risk, in which case "Mean" expresses a rate. With a divisor of 1, you get the Poisson confidence interval for a count.

10.6   Immediate commands

Immediate commands do not use the data in memory; instead, you enter the data with the command (see [U] **19 Immediate commands**). Typically, you will want to perform some calculations on tabular information. Immediate commands end with i, e.g., tabi, ttesti, and cii (but not all commands that end with i are immediate commands). cii was demonstrated in section 10.5. The following sections show the command syntax, but you might prefer to use the dialogs, e.g.,

```
. db tabi
```

tabi

tabi is the immediate form of tab2, and you can use the same options. Say that you saw the following table in a paper but suspected that the reported Pr < 0.05 was misleading because of small numbers:

Treatment	Died	Survived	Total
A	4	10	14
B	7	3	10
Total	11	13	24

$$\chi^2 = 4.03; \; df = 1; \; Pr < 0.05$$

In tabi, you entered the data for each row, separated by \ (backslash):

```
. tabi 4 10 \ 7 3, chi exact
```

	col		
row	1	2	Total
1	4	10	14
2	7	3	10
Total	11	13	24

```
          Pearson chi2(1) =    4.0328   Pr = 0.045
             Fisher's exact =              0.095
     1-sided Fisher's exact =              0.055
```

Fisher's exact test gave Pr = 0.09, so your suspicion was right.

Immediate epitab commands

The immediate epitab commands (see [ST] **epitab**) make unstratified analyses only. For help in interpreting the output, see sections 12.1, 12.2, and 14.1.

iri is the immediate form of ir (incidence-rate ratio, incidence-rate difference). The arguments must be entered in the correct order, as illustrated below.

	Exposed	Unexposed
Events	17	23
Time at risk	231.5	196.4

```
. iri 17 23 231.5 196.4
```

	Exposed	Unexposed	Total		
Cases	17	23	40		
Person-time	231.5	196.4	427.9		
Incidence Rate	.0734341	.1171079	.0934798		
	Point estimate		[95% Conf. Interval]		
Inc. rate diff.	-.0436738		-.1029115	.0155639	
Inc. rate ratio	.6270636		.3144679	1.226403	(exact)
Prev. frac. ex.	.3729364		-.2264033	.6855321	(exact)
Prev. frac. pop	.2017639				

```
                (midp)   Pr(k<=17) =                    0.0731   (exact)
                (midp) 2*Pr(k<=17) =                    0.1463   (exact)
```

csi is the immediate form of cs (risk ratio, risk difference):

	Exposed	Unexposed
Event	7	12
No event	19	21

```
. csi 7 12 19 21
```

cci is the immediate form of cc (odds ratio). The arguments are the same as those in csi:

```
. cci 7 12 19 21
```

ttesti

ttesti is the immediate form of ttest. You input number of observations, mean, and SD for each group:

```
. ttesti 32 1.35 .27 50 1.77 .33
```

display: Stata as a pocket calculator

The display command gives you the opportunity to perform calculations not involving the data in memory; see [R] **display**:

```
. display 2*c(pi)*7
43.982297
```

You can include explanatory text:

```
. display "The circumference of a circle with radius 7 is " 2*c(pi)*7
The circumference of a circle with radius 7 is 43.982297
```

c(pi) is a Stata constant. c() contains system parameters, settings, and constants; see section 17.1. You can display them by typing

```
. creturn list
```

With display you can use the built-in functions, e.g., to find a *p*-value from a chi-squared test:

```
. display chi2tail(1,3.84)
.05004352
```

For more information, see the functions available in [D] **functions** or type

```
. help functions
```

11 Graphs

Stata's graphics system is powerful. You can often create desired graphs with a simple command or a few clicks in a dialog box. Preparing a publication-ready graph may require more effort. Some graphic programs allow you to use the mouse to modify the elements of a graph directly; Stata does not, but you can build a command that allows you to have full control over the looks of the graph. Much of this chapter deals with this issue.

Look at the illustrations in this chapter to get some ideas of the types of graphs available in Stata. At http://www.ats.ucla.edu/stat/stata/Library/GraphExamples/, you find several graph examples with the commands used. The *Graphics Reference Manual* ([G]) gives more examples and is included in Stata's Complete Documentation Set. *A Visual Guide to Stata Graphics* (Mitchell 2004) is also accessible and full of examples.

The main graph types described in the *Graphics Reference Manual* are

```
graph bar
graph box
graph dot
graph matrix
graph pie
graph twoway
```

In `graph twoway`, there are several plot types available, such as `twoway scatter` and `twoway line`.

Besides these graph types, there are others, described in [R], such as `histogram` and `dotplot`, and there are graph types related to other topics, such as survival analysis, described in [ST], e.g., `sts graph`.

This chapter shows a full do-file for most graphs. Some of the other chapters show graphs, but only with the minimum commands needed to display them in close to final form. The full do-files for all graphs are, however, available at this book's web site: http://www.stata-press.com/books/ishr.html.

11.1   Anatomy of a graph

Figure 11.1 shows the most important elements of a graph. The *graph* area is the entire figure, including everything in the graph, while the *plot* area is the central part of the graph, defined by the axes.

A graph consists of several elements: title, legend, axes, and one or more plots, for example, two scatterplots within the same plot area. Figure 11.1 includes two scatterplots.

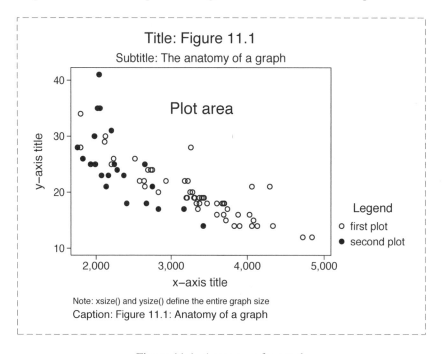

Figure 11.1: Anatomy of a graph

There are two types of elements in a graph like figure 11.1. The *plot* elements are the dots in the two scatterplots. The *graph* elements are all the rest: axes, titles, legend, etc. This distinction is reflected in the syntax, as you will see in section 11.2. Below is the do-file that generated figure 11.1. Most elements of this complex command for a complex graph will be explained later.

```
                        ──────── gph_fig11_1.do ────────
* gph_fig11_1.do

sysuse auto.dta, clear
set scheme lean1

* see section 11.2 for explanation of command listed below
*
twoway                                                      /// G
  (scatter mpg weight if foreign==0)                        /// P
  (scatter mpg weight if foreign==1)                        /// P
  ,                                                         ///
  title("Title: Figure 11.1")                               /// G
  subtitle("Subtitle: The anatomy of a graph")              /// G
  ytitle("y-axis title") xtitle("x-axis title")             /// G
  legend(title("Legend", size(*0.8))                        /// G
    order(1 "first plot" 2 "second plot"))                  /// G
  note("Note: xsize() and ysize() define the entire graph size") /// G
  caption("Caption: Figure 11.1: Anatomy of a graph")       /// G
  text(35 3400 "Plot area", size(*1.5))                     /// G
  graphregion(lpattern(dash) lcolor(black) lwidth(*0.5))    /// G
  xsize(4.4) ysize(3.3)
```

11.2 Anatomy of graph commands

Overall command structure

The general syntax of a graph command is

    graph-command (*plottype*, *plot-options*) (*plottype*, *plot-options*), *graph-options*

In the command generating figure 11.1, `twoway` is the graph type, and `scatter` is a plot type. The syntax above is the syntax style generated by the dialogs, and this book will follow it. You may see another less transparent syntax style, putting bars (||) where the standard syntax has a right parenthesis closing a plot type specification:

    graph-command plottype, *plot-options* || *plottype*, *plot-options* ||, *graph-options*

The comma separating the plot specifications from the graph options is important. In the do-file that generates figure 11.1, the P and G comments tell whether a command element is a plot specification or a graph option. In complex commands, the pivotal comma has a line of its own, just for clarity (Stata does not care).

This section will show parts of commands like this:

```
. ..., title("74 car makes")
. twoway (scatter mpg weight, msymbol(Oh)), ...
```

In the first line, `title()` is a graph option; it is preceded by the pivotal comma. In the second line, any graph options can follow after the pivotal comma; `msymbol()` is a plot option, not a graph option.

The full command for a scatterplot is something like

```
. graph twoway (scatter mpg weight), ...
```

but it may have this shorter form, which is the syntax generated by the dialogs,

```
. twoway (scatter mpg weight), ...
```

and Stata also understands the following short version:

```
. scatter mpg weight
```

Options

Graph commands may have options; as in other Stata commands, a comma precedes the options. `title()` is an option to the `twoway` graph command:

```
. twoway (scatter mpg weight), title("74 car makes")
```

Plot types may have options. `msymbol()` is an option to `scatter` and is located within the parentheses delimiting the plot specification. `msymbol(Oh)` selects a hollow circle as the marker symbol:

```
. twoway (scatter mpg weight, msymbol(Oh)), ...
```

Options can have suboptions. `size()` is a suboption to the `title()` graph option; here it sets the title text size to 80% of the default size:

```
. ..., title("74 car makes", size(*0.8))
```

The sequence of options makes no difference.

> **Warning:** Options in principle do not allow a space between the option keyword and its parenthesis, like the following ($\square$ denotes a space):
>
> ```
> . ..., title□("74 car makes")
> ```
>
> The error message may be confusing, such as "Unmatched quotes" or "Option not allowed".

> **Advice:** Graph commands tend to include a lot of nested parentheses, and you may make errors (I often do). In the Do-file Editor, you can place the cursor within parentheses and press *Ctrl-B* (B for balance) to see the matching parentheses.

Variable lists: Long and wide data formats

Most two-way plot types have one or more dependent y-variables and one independent x-variable, so the scatterplot syntax can be written

>   . **twoway (scatter** *yvarlist xvar*, *plot_options*)**,** *graph_options*

The uslifeexp.dta dataset accompanying Stata includes data on U.S. life expectancy for each year from 1900 to 1999 for the whole nation (le), for males (le_male), for white males (le_wmale), etc. A graph from these data is shown in figure 11.31, section 11.8. See the variables in the dataset with describe:

```
. sysuse uslifeexp.dta
(U.S. life expectancy, 1900-1999)

. describe

Contains data from C:\Stata\ado\base\u\uslifeexp.dta
  obs:           100                          U.S. life expectancy, 1900-1999
  vars:           10                          30 Mar 2005 04:31
  size:         4,200 (99.9% of memory free)  (_dta has notes)
```

variable name	storage type	display format	value label	variable label
year	int	%9.0g		Year
le	float	%9.0g		life expectancy
(output omitted)				
le_wmale	float	%9.0g		Life expectancy, white males
le_wfemale	float	%9.0g		Life expectancy, white females
(output omitted)				
le_bmale	float	%9.0g		Life expectancy, black males
le_bfemale	float	%9.0g		Life expectancy, black females

```
Sorted by:  year
```

The data structure is "wide"; for each observation (a year) there is information on results for subgroups of the population; for white and black males and females it looks like this:

```
. list year le_wmale le_wfemale le_bmale le_bfemale if year<1903,
> abbrev(10)
```

	year	le_wmale	le_wfemale	le_bmale	le_bfemale
1.	1900	46.6	48.7	32.5	33.5
2.	1901	48	51	32.2	35.3
3.	1902	50.2	53.8	32.9	36.4

The corresponding "long" structure, with one observation for each year, sex, and race group, would look like this:

```
. list year le sex race if year<1903, sepby(sex race)
```

	year	le	sex	race
1.	1900	46.6	1	1
2.	1901	48	1	1
3.	1902	50.2	1	1
101.	1900	48.7	2	1
102.	1901	51	2	1
103.	1902	53.8	2	1
201.	1900	32.5	1	2
202.	1901	32.2	1	2
203.	1902	32.9	1	2
301.	1900	33.5	2	2
302.	1901	35.3	2	2
303.	1902	36.4	2	2

With a wide data structure, the command to plot a line for each sex and race group is

```
. twoway (line le_wmale le_wfemale le_bmale le_bfemale year), ...
```

With a long data structure, the command gets more complex (best suited for a do-file):

```
. twoway (line le year if sex==1 & race==1)    ///
    (line le year if sex==2 & race==1)    ///
    (line le year if sex==1 & race==2)    ///
    (line le year if sex==2 & race==2)    ///
    , ...
```

In the graph examples, section 11.8, I show examples of both structures. The reshape command (see section 9.6) is a tool for transforming between long and wide data structures.

11.3   Graph size

The twoway scatter command creates scatterplots. Figure 11.2 is the default appearance with the s2mono scheme (for more about schemes, see section 11.4):

```
. sysuse auto.dta, clear
(1978 Automobile Data)
. set scheme s2mono
. twoway (scatter mpg weight)
```

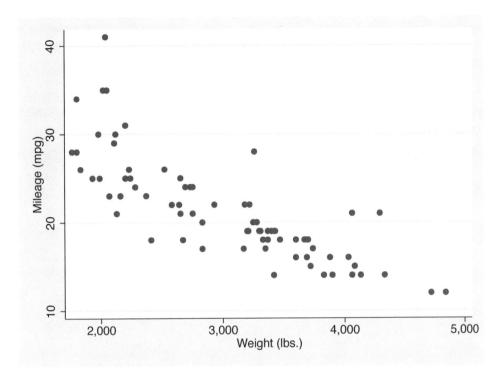

Figure 11.2: Default size of a graph under the s2mono scheme

If you find figure 11.2 too large, you can reduce the size with the xsize() and ysize() graph options, which determine the size of the entire graph area. The arguments are in inches:

```
. twoway (scatter mpg weight), xsize(3) ysize(2.2)
```

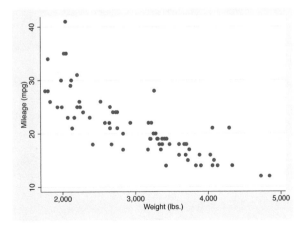

Figure 11.3: Reduced-size graph, marker and text size reduced proportionally

Now the size is right, but the text and marker size shrank with the graph; in particular, the text is too small. To enlarge marker and text size, use the `scale()` graph option; in figure 11.4, text and markers are enlarged by 40%:

```
. twoway (scatter mpg weight), xsize(3) ysize(2.2) scale(1.4)
```

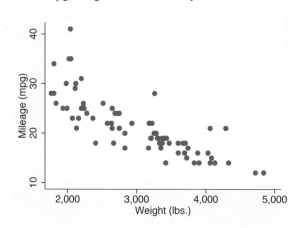

Figure 11.4: Change marker and text size with the `scale()` option

As you will see in section 11.7, you can also modify the size of individual graph and plot elements.

The `xsize()` and `ysize()` options determine the entire graph size, not only the plot area. To control the aspect ratio (the y/x ratio) of the plot area directly, use the `aspectratio()` option. In figure 11.5, say that we wanted a square plot area:

```
. twoway (scatter mpg weight), xsize(3) ysize(2.2) scale(1.4)
> aspectratio(1)
```

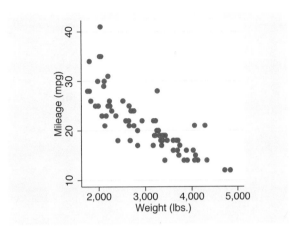

Figure 11.5: Controlling the plot area aspect ratio with the `aspectratio()` option

11.4   Schemes

Figures 11.2–11.5 used the s2mono scheme with a shaded background and faint grid lines. There are other schemes, such as s1color and s1mono; they have no shaded background and no grid lines, but they have a full frame around the plot area:

```
. set scheme s1mono
. twoway (scatter mpg weight), xsize(3) ysize(2.2) scale(1.4)
```

(Continued on next page)

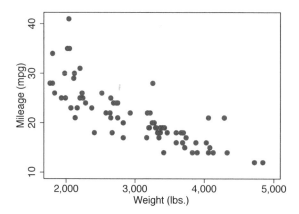

Figure 11.6: s1mono scheme has no grid lines but has a framed plot area.

Two other schemes are lean1 and lean2 (Juul 2003). They avoid colors and grayscales, keeping most things black and white. The lean schemes are not part of official Stata, but you can find and install them by typing

```
. findit lean schemes
```

Style is partly a matter of taste, but it also depends on what you are going to use the graphs for. For a slide show, carefully using colors can be of great value, but colors and grayscales can cause problems when photocopying, and many scientific journals require that you submit lean black and white graphs.

Figure 11.7 displays the same information as figure 11.6 but with the `lean2` scheme:

```
. set scheme lean2
. twoway (scatter mpg weight), xsize(3) ysize(2.2) scale(1.4)
```

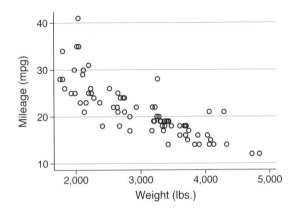

Figure 11.7: Scheme `lean2`

Like s2color and s2mono, the `lean2` scheme has horizontal grid lines. Like s1color and s1mono, the `lean1` scheme has no grid lines but has a full frame around the plot area:

```
. set scheme lean1
. twoway (scatter mpg weight), xsize(3) ysize(2.2) scale(1.4)
```

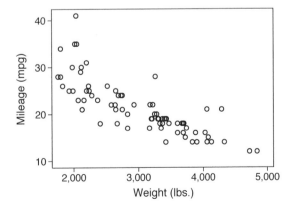

Figure 11.8: Scheme `lean1`

A scheme defines the defaults, but it does not prevent you from making modifications. You might want a blue triangle as a marker (see section 11.7 on marker options):

```
. twoway (scatter mpg weight, msymbol(T) mcolor(blue)), ...
```

or even a triangle with a blue outline and a red fill:

```
. twoway (scatter mpg weight, ms(T) mlcolor(blue) mfcolor(red)), ...
```

To make a scheme (for example, lean1) your default, type

```
. set scheme lean1, permanently
```

To see a list of the schemes installed on your computer, use the command

```
. graph query, schemes
```

A Visual Guide to Stata Graphics (Mitchell 2004) demonstrates several colorful schemes; they may be useful, e.g., for slide shows. To install the schemes, type

```
. net from http://www.stata-press.com/data/vgsg
. net install vgsg
```

Read more about schemes in the *Graphics Manual*, starting with [G] **schemes**.

11.5   Graph options: Axes

Now things get a bit more complicated. Any command can be given from the command line, but it is easier and safer to build complex commands in do-files; chances are you will need to modify your first attempt. I begin the name of do-files defining graphs with a gph prefix for easy identification, and I begin each do-file with a comment indicating the do-file's own name. I also always include a use command (or, as here, a sysuse) to indicate the dataset.

Axis labels, ticks, and grid lines

Stata sets reasonable ticks and labels at the axes; you can also define them yourself. The following command sets a tick and a label for every 25 years at the x-axis; minor ticks divide each major interval into 5-year segments. The y-axis label definition had no consequences; Stata would have chosen these values anyway. Label specifications follow the rules for numeric lists; see section 4.3.

```
─────────────────────── gph_fig11_9.do ───────────────────────
* gph_fig11_9.do

sysuse uslifeexp.dta, clear
set scheme lean2

twoway (line le year)                 ///
  ,                                   ///
  xlabel(1900(25)2000)  xmtick(##5)   ///
  ylabel(40(10)80)                    ///
  xsize(3.1) ysize(2.2) scale(1.4)
```

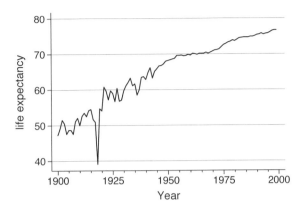

Figure 11.9: Specifying *x*-axis labels and ticks explicitly

You can turn grid lines on and off; the following command turns off horizontal and turns on vertical grid lines:

```
                              ───── gph_fig11_10.do ─────
* gph_fig11_10.do

sysuse uslifeexp.dta, clear
set scheme lean2

twoway (line le year)              ///
  ,                                ///
  xlabel(1900(20)2000, grid)       ///
  ylabel(, nogrid)                 ///
  xsize(3.1) ysize(2.2) scale(1.4)
```

(Continued on next page)

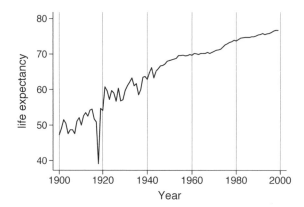

Figure 11.10: Turning horizontal grid lines off and vertical grid lines on

By definition, the axes in two-way graphs are continuous, but categorical variables may be used. To display value labels rather than codes, use the `valuelabel` suboption, as in figure 11.32. The ticks were turned off, too:

> . ..., `xlabel(1(1)8, valuelabel noticks)`

Tick labels can also be specified explicitly in the label option. To include a leading zero in the y-axis labels in figure 11.12, the `ylabel()` option was used:

> . ..., `ylabel(.1 "0.1" 1 10 100)`

In the `s1` and `s2` schemes the y-axis labels by default are vertically oriented. If you want horizontal y-axis labels (as in the `lean` schemes) with an `s1` or `s2` scheme, type

> . ..., `ylabel(, angle(0))`

To remove labels and ticks from the x-axis, as in figure 11.33, type

> . ..., `xlabel(none)`

To hide the y-axis, as in figure 11.33, use

> . ..., `yscale(off)`

You may expand an axis beyond what the data require by defining a value range, as in figure 11.32:

> . ..., `xscale(range(0.5 8.5))`

Most graphs by default leave some space (the plot region margin) between axes and the closest plot values, but in figure 11.11, we want the x-axis to start at zero. You can do this by using the `plotregion(margin(l=0))` option (l for left, r for right, t for top, b for bottom). If you want all margins to be zero, the option is `plotregion(margin(zero))`.

If you want to display decimal commas rather than periods, use the Stata command

```
. set dp comma
```

and return to the default decimal period by typing

```
. set dp period
```

Log-scaled axes

You can use log scales; a detailed axis-label specification is often required, as in figure 11.11. By default, there would be too many horizontal grid lines; they were turned off by `ylabel()`'s `nogrid` option, and four thin reference lines were drawn by `yline()` instead.

```
────────────── gph_fig11_11.do ──────────────
* gph_fig11_11.do

cd C:\docs\ishr
use agemort.dta, clear
set scheme lean2

twoway (line mort age)                              ///
  ,                                                 ///
  plotregion(margin(l=0))                           ///
  yscale(log)                                       ///
  ylabel(.1 .2 .5 1 2 5 10 20 50 100 200 500, nogrid)  ///
  yline(0.1 1 10 100, lwidth(*0.5))                 ///
  xsize(3.1) ysize(2.2) scale(1.4)
```

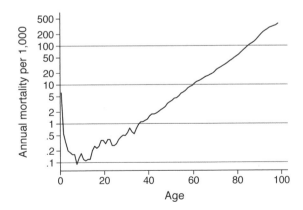

Figure 11.11: Log-scaled *y*-axis

In figure 11.11, there are probably too many *y*-axis labels; figure 11.12 shows another principle for putting labels and ticks on a log-scaled axis, using `ymticks()` (minor ticks):

```
―――――――――――――― gph_fig11_12.eps ――――――――――――――
* gph_fig11_12.do

cd C:\docs\ishr
use agemort.dta, clear
set scheme lean2

twoway (line mort age)                                    ///
  ,                                                       ///
  plotregion(margin(l=0))                                 ///
  yscale(log)                                             ///
  ylabel(.1 "0.1" 1 10 100)                               ///
  ymticks(.2(.1).9  2(1)9  20(10)90  200(100)500)         ///
  xsize(3.1) ysize(2.2) scale(1.4)
```

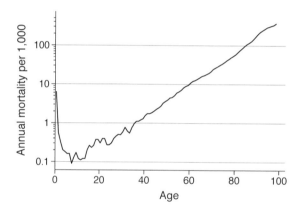

Figure 11.12: Log scaled y-axis; alternative labeling

Multiple axes

You can have more than one x- and one y-axis. Figure 11.13, reconstructed from Doll and Hill (1950), has two y-axes, one for lung cancer mortality and one for cigarette consumption. The original information about pounds of tobacco was recalculated to grams (1 cigarette = 1 g):

```
                            ─── gph_fig11_13.do ───
* gph_fig11_13.do

set scheme lean1

clear
input year tobacco cancer
1900  .4   .5
1907  .7   .6
1912  .9   1.0
1924 1.9   1.9
1930 2.4   4.0
1936 2.8   7.5
1947 4.2  22.5
end

generate cigarettes = 454*tobacco          // (1 lb. = 454 grams)

twoway                                                         ///
  (line cancer year, yaxis(1) lpattern(l))                     ///
  (line cigarettes year, yaxis(2) lpattern(dash))              ///
  ,                                                            ///
  xtitle("Year")                                               ///
  ytitle("Annual lung cancer" "mortality per 100,000", axis(1))   ///
  ytitle("Cigarettes per person per year", axis(2))            ///
  legend(order(2 "Cigarette consumption" 1 "Lung cancer mortality")) ///
  plotregion(margin(b=0))                                      ///
  xsize(5) ysize(2) aspectratio(0.75) scale(1.4)
```

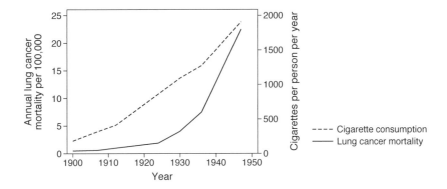

Figure 11.13: Graph with two *y*-axes

In the plot specifications, the axes are referred to as yaxis(1) and yaxis(2); in the ytitle() options, they are referred to as axis(1) and axis(2).

11.6 Graph options: Text elements

Titles and texts

Graph title and subtitle, axis titles, notes, and captions are defined as shown in figure 11.1. By default, axis titles use variable labels if they are defined, otherwise they use variable names.

You can define a two-line text by (see example figure 11.13) typing

```
. ..., ytitle("Annual lung cancer" "mortality per 100,000")
```

Legends

Say that we want to put two scatterplots—one for domestic and one for foreign cars—in one graph. We start with the s1mono scheme:

```
––––––––––––––––––––––––––––––– gph_fig11_14.do –––––––––––––––––
* gph_fig11_14.do

sysuse auto.dta, clear
set scheme s1mono

twoway                                        ///
  (scatter mpg weight if foreign==0)          ///
  (scatter mpg weight if foreign==1)          ///
  ,                                           ///
  xsize(3.1) ysize(2.2) scale(1.4)
```

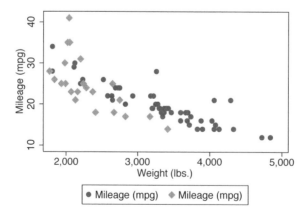

Figure 11.14: Two plots in one graph generate a legend—but this one is useless.

If there is more than one plot in a graph, the legend is used to explain the meaning of the various marker and line styles. In figure 11.14, the legend does not display the information we need; to get it right, we must include a `legend()` option in the `twoway` command.

You might also find that the two gray-scaled symbols in figure 11.14 are too indistinct. One option is to define the symbols explicitly (see section 11.7); another is to see what the `lean` schemes do. Here you can also put a title for the legend in figure 11.15:

```
────────────────────────── gph_fig11_15.do ──────────
* gph_fig11_15.do

sysuse auto.dta, clear
set scheme lean1

twoway                                                     ///
  (scatter mpg weight if foreign==0)                       ///
  (scatter mpg weight if foreign==1)                       ///
  ,                                                        ///
  legend(title("Origin") order(1 "Domestic" 2 "Foreign")) ///
  xsize(3.1) ysize(2.2) scale(1.4)
```

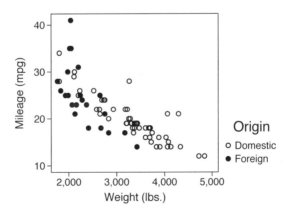

Figure 11.15: `lean` schemes provide distinct markers, but legend placement distorts plot area.

You now see more distinct symbols, but the graph became distorted—why? Whereas the `s1` and `s2` schemes put the legend below the x-axis, the `lean` schemes put it to the right of the plot area. The `xsize()` and `ysize()` options define the size of the entire graph, including axis titles, labels, and the legend. To compensate, `xsize()` must be increased; 3.8 inches seems to work. We also reduce the size of the legend title:

```
———————————————————— gph_fig11_16.do ————————————————————
* gph_fig11_16.do

sysuse auto.dta, clear
set scheme lean1

twoway                                          ///
  (scatter mpg weight if foreign==0)            ///
  (scatter mpg weight if foreign==1)            ///
  ,                                             ///
  legend(title("Origin", size(*0.8))            ///
    order(1 "Domestic" 2 "Foreign"))            ///
  xsize(3.8) ysize(2.2) scale(1.4)
```

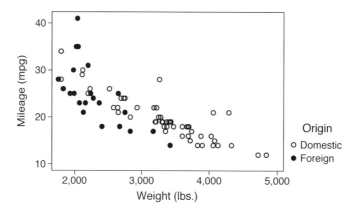

Figure 11.16: Distorted plot area corrected by increasing xsize()

Instead of experimenting with xsize() and ysize() to obtain the desired plot aspect ratio, you may use the aspectratio() option. Be generous with the xsize() option, and use aspectratio() to control the y/x ratio of the plot area (it looks exactly like figure 11.16):

    . ..., xsize(4) ysize(2.2) scale(1.4) aspectratio(0.7)

Placing text elements

The placement of text elements, such as titles and the legend, is defined by location relative to the plot area (*ring* position) and a direction (*clock* position); see [G] ***title_options***. The placement of elements in figure 11.1 was determined by the scheme applied (lean1); the placements are shown in table 11.1. The only difference from the s1 and s2 schemes is the legend placement; they put the legend at pos(6).

Table 11.1: Placement of text elements with the lean schemes

Element	Ring position ring()	Clock position pos()	Position can be modified?
Plot area	0	...	No
y-axis title	1	9	No
x-axis title	1	6	No
Title	7	12	Yes
Subtitle	6	12	Yes
Legend	3	4	Yes
Note	4	7	Yes
Caption	5	7	Yes

The details of the outer rings are hardly interesting to most users, but specifying ring(0) places an object within the plot area. To place the legend in the upper-right corner, specify the two o'clock position by pos(2):

```
─────────────── gph_fig11_17.do ───────────────
* gph_fig11_17.do

sysuse auto.dta, clear
set scheme lean1

twoway                                                    ///
  (scatter mpg weight if foreign==0)                      ///
  (scatter mpg weight if foreign==1)                      ///
  ,                                                        ///
  legend(order(1 "Domestic" 2 "Foreign") ring(0) pos(2))  ///
  xsize(3.1) ysize(2.2) scale(1.4)
```

(Continued on next page)

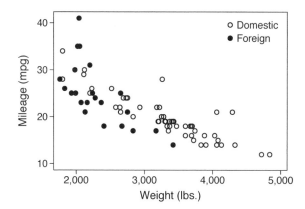

Figure 11.17: Legend placed inside plot area by the `ring(0)` argument

You can put a text block anywhere in the plot area by specifying its y and x coordinates; `place(0)` (the default) means that the coordinates apply to the center of the text block; `place(8)` that the text is placed at eight o'clock relative to the point defined by the coordinates. `place(sw)` means the same as `place(8)`. See the example in figure 11.1:

```
. ..., text(35 3400 "Plot area", place(0))
```

but since `place(0)` is the default, this suboption could have been omitted.

11.7 Plot options: Markers, lines, etc.

Stata chooses markers, line styles, etc., from a style list, which depends on the scheme selected. I recommend that you run the first version of a `graph` command without specifying marker or line options and then modify them if you need to do that.

Table 11.2 shows the options and their arguments for markers, bars, and lines; examples of their use are shown in the following table.

Table 11.2: Options for defining the appearance of lines, bars, markers, etc.

All elements, except markers		Markers	
Overall color:	color()	Overall color:	mcolor()
Fill color:	fcolor()	Fill color:	mfcolor()
Line, outline color:	lcolor()	Outline color:	mlcolor()
Line, outline width:	lwidth()	Outline width:	mlwidth()
Line, outline pattern:	lpattern()	Marker symbol:	msymbol()
		Marker size:	msize()

Bars, areas, textboxes, etc., have an outline and a fill that may be defined separately, e.g., by using lcolor() to specify the outline color and fcolor() to specify the fill color. Marker options all start with m; mlcolor() defines the marker outline color, mfcolor() the marker fill color.

Colors

To see a list of the colors available, use the command

```
. help colorstyle
```

To see one color, e.g., lavender, on the screen, type

```
. palette color lavender
```

If you installed the schemes related to *A Visual Guide to Stata Graphics* (see section 11.4), the following command will display a full color palette:

```
. vgcolormap
```

Gray colors have names from gs0 (black) to gs16 (white). For an example how to use gray colors for bar fills, see figure 11.27:

```
. ..., bar(3, fcolor(gs9))
```

When printing or photocopying graphs with colors or gray scales, look carefully at the result; the appearance is sensitive to printer setup, toner quality, etc. For more on this topic, see section 11.10.

Lines

You can see most of the available line patterns by typing

```
. palette linepalette
```

Figure 11.18 shows a modified palette of the patterns.

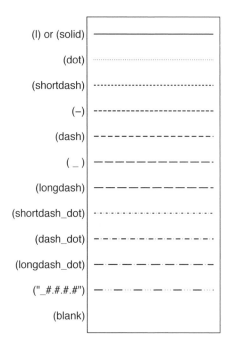

Figure 11.18: Line patterns

Besides using the patterns created by Stata, you may create your own by a formula, e.g,

```
. twoway (line le year, lpattern("_#.#.#.#")), ...
```

where # puts a little extra space between the elements.

The main use of line patterns is with connecting line plots (the `lpattern()` option); you can see an example in figure 11.31, but you may also use it for, e.g., bar outlines.

A scheme has a default sequence of line patterns to be used; you can see an example of this in figure 11.30. We found the default pattern sequence to be less than optimal here, so we modified it in figure 11.31.

Marker symbols

Figure 11.19 shows the marker symbols used for scatterplots, etc. It was created by typing

```
. palette symbolpalette
```

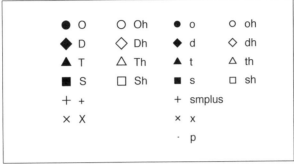

(symbols shown at larger than default size)

Figure 11.19: Marker symbols

To define a hollow circle, you type

```
. twoway (scatter mpg weight, msymbol(Oh)), ...
```

A hollow circle (Oh) is transparent. You can obtain a circle with a nontransparent white fill by typing

```
. twoway (scatter mpg weight, msymbol(O) mfcolor(white)), ...
```

A scheme has a default sequence of markers. The s1 and s2 schemes also vary the marker colors, whereas the lean schemes keep all markers black. A scheme defines the defaults, but it does not prevent you from making modifications. You might want a blue triangle as the marker

```
. twoway (scatter mpg weight, msymbol(T) mcolor(blue)), ...
```

or even a triangle with a blue outline and a red fill:

```
. twoway (scatter mpg weight, ms(T) mlcolor(blue) mfcolor(red)), ...
```

For more examples of markers, see figures 11.28 and 11.29.

Modifying size of elements

The width of a line is controlled by the lwidth() option, as in

```
. twoway (line le year, lpattern(dash) lwidth(*0.8)), ...
```

making the line width 80% of the default; see an example in figure 11.31.

The size of a marker is controlled by the `msize()` option, as in

```
. twoway (scatter mpg weight, msymbol(Th) msize(*1.5)), ...
```

making the marker size 50% larger than the default; for an example, see figure 11.28.

As shown in section 11.3, the `scale()` option lets you modify the size of many elements at once (e.g., texts, symbol sizes).

11.8   Graph examples

Here you will find illustrations of some important graph types, including the commands that generated the graphs. The appearance is different from the manual's graphs; it comes from the *schemes* `lean1` and `lean2`, described in section 11.4.

I will show the do-file used to make each graph, including the data for the graph or a `use` command. I suggest giving do-files that generate graphs a gph prefix for easy identification.

Histograms

A histogram illustrates the distribution of a continuous variable; see [R] **histogram**. Figure 11.20 shows the weight distribution of 74 car makes. If you do not specify the number of bars (or number of bins, as it is often called in a histogram context), the placement of the first bar, or the width of bars, Stata will decided these for you:

```
―――――――――――――― gph_fig11_20.do ――――――――――――――
* gph_fig11_20.do

sysuse auto.dta, clear
set scheme lean2

histogram weight, xsize(3.1) ysize(2.2) scale(1.4)
```

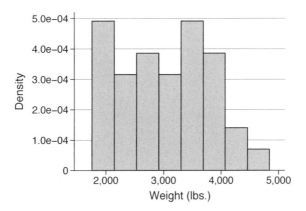

Figure 11.20: Histogram

The look of figure 11.20 is not quite satisfactory, so let's make some modifications: we want to have bars reflect "natural" 500-pound groups (the start() and width() options). The *y*-axis displays the density; we want the number of observations (the frequency option). We also want a normal curve and a kernel density curve overlaid (the normal and kdensity options):

```
─────────────────────── gph_fig11_21.do ───────────────────────
* gph_fig11_21.do

sysuse auto.dta, clear
set scheme lean2

histogram weight                ///
  ,                             ///
  frequency                     ///
  normal                        ///
  kdensity                      ///
  start(1000) width(500)        ///
  xsize(3.1) ysize(2.2) scale(1.4)
```

(Continued on next page)

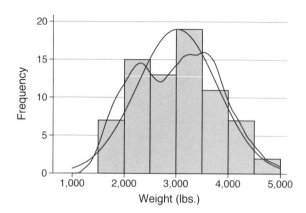

Figure 11.21: Histogram with a normal and a kernel density curve overlaid

It is striking that the shapes of the histograms in figure 11.20 and 11.21 are so different. With few observations, varying the cutpoints between bins can make quite a difference in appearance. The kernel density curve can be considered a smoothed version of a histogram (for more information, see [R] **kdensity**); here it suggests that the cars consist of two subpopulations (which is actually the case; look at figure 11.23 or try to make separate histograms for foreign and domestic cars).

Boxplots and dotplots

In a box-and-whisker plot, the box displays the interquartile range (the 25th–75th percentiles) and the median (see [G] **graph box**). The whiskers display the upper and lower values within 1.5 times the interquartile range beyond the 25th and 75th percentile. Any outliers beyond that get their own marker. In figure 11.22, the orientation is horizontal and is obtained by the graph hbox command; graph box gives a vertical orientation. The value labels in figure 11.22 are less than optimal; see figure 11.26 for instructions on how to modify them. For the over() option, see bar graphs later this section.

```
                        ──────── gph_fig11_22.do ────────
* gph_fig11_22.do

cd C:\docs\ishr
use lbw1.dta, clear
set scheme lean2

graph hbox bwt                  ///
   ,                            ///
   over(smoke) over(race)       ///
   xsize(3.8) ysize(2.2) scale(1.4)
```

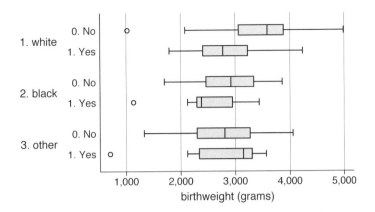

Figure 11.22: Horizontal box plot

A dot plot can be used for similar purposes; it can be considered a kind of a histogram (see [R] **dotplot**). dotplot is described in the *Base Reference Manual*; it is different from the plot type described in [G] **graph dot**. In figure 11.23, the center option makes the columns symmetrical; the nx() option sets the horizontal dot density, and the ny() option sets the number of bins. You might need to experiment to get a satisfactory result. msymbol(O) defines the marker symbol as a filled circle.

```
                                   gph_fig11_23.do
* gph_fig11_23.do

sysuse auto.dta, clear
set scheme lean1

dotplot weight                    ///
  ,                               ///
  over(foreign) center msymbol(O) ///
  nx(14) ny(20)                   ///
  xsize(2.8) ysize(2.2) scale(1.4)
```

(Continued on next page)

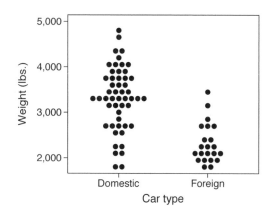

Figure 11.23: Dotplot

Bar graphs

Bar graphs typically show the distribution of a quantity (count, sum, mean) over groups defined by one or more categorical variables (see [G] **graph bar**).

The main elements in the graph bar command are

> . **graph bar** (*stat*) *yvarlist* [(*stat*) *yvarlist*], **over**(*xvar*) [**over**(*xvar*)]
> *other_options*

(*stat*) can be, e.g.,

(asis)   the values as they are (one observation per group, as in figure 11.24)

(mean)   mean of values in a group (the default)

(count) number of valid observations in a group

(*stat*) can be any of the statistics available in collapse; see [D] **collapse** or type

> . **help collapse**

The over() option defines the groups to be displayed. The graph hbar command gives horizontal bars.

Figure 11.24 illustrates the prevalence of diabetes; data are entered in wide form:

```
─────────────────────────── gph_fig11_24.do ───────────────────────────
* gph_fig11_24.do

clear
input str5 age diabm diabf
16-24   .9   .2
25-44   .8   .8
45-66  3.8  2.9
67-79  8.2  5.4
80+    9.1  7.2
end

set scheme lean2

graph bar (asis) diabm diabf              ///
  ,                                       ///
  over(age)                               ///
  b1title("Age")                          ///
  ytitle("Prevalence (per cent)")         ///
  legend(order(1 "Males" 2 "Females"))    ///
  blabel(bar, format(%03.1f))             ///
  xsize(4.4) ysize(2.2) scale(1.4)
```

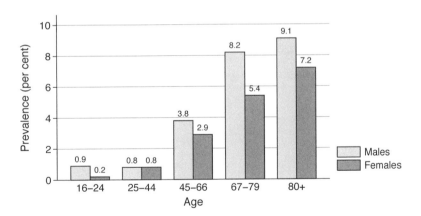

Figure 11.24: Bar graph constructed from tabular data

There are two *y*-variables in the *yvarlist* (diabm and diabf); the statistic (asis) corresponds to one observation per group. The default statistic is (mean), and with one observation per group, a value and its mean are the same; so the command could have been

. `graph bar (mean) diabm diabf, ...`

and even, since (`mean`) is the default statistic,

> . `graph bar diabm diabf, ...`

For some reason, the `xtitle()` option is not valid for bar graphs. To generate an *x*-axis title, you can, however, use `b1title()` instead.

The `blabel()` option lets you put labels on top of the bars; `format(%03.1f)` displays leading zeros. Actually, I prefer to avoid such labels, but here you saw how to make them.

Bar fill colors (see table 11.2) are assigned automatically according to the scheme. The following option would generate a dark fill for females:

> . `..., bar(2, fcolor(gs3))`

The `lbw1.dta` dataset is in long format. The `over()` option may be nested to three layers; figure 11.25 has two layers:

```
——————————————— gph_fig11_25.do ———————————————
* gph_fig11_25.do

cd C:\docs\ishr
use lbw1.dta, clear
set scheme lean2

graph bar (mean) bwt                    ///
  ,                                      ///
  over(smoke) over(race)                ///
  xsize(3.3) ysize(2.2) scale(1.4)
```

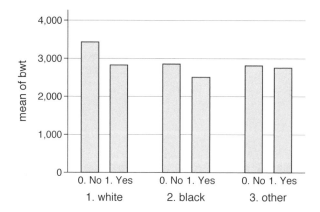

Figure 11.25: Bar graph nested to two layers

The bars are labeled according to the value labels in the dataset; they are, however, poor labels, and I must redefine the value labels before using the `graph` command. Figure 11.26 shows improved titles and labels. It also shows how the `asyvars` option may be used to restructure the graph: it behaves as if the data were in wide format with two y-variables (birthweight among smokers and nonsmokers) and the command had one `over(race)` option:

```
———————————————— gph_fig11_26.do ————————————————
* gph_fig11_26.do

cd C:\docs\ishr
use lbw1.dta, clear
set scheme lean2

label define yesno 0 "Nonsmokers" 1 "Smokers", modify
label define race 1 "Whites" 2 "Blacks" 3 "Others", modify

graph bar (mean) bwt                    ///
  ,                                     ///
  over(smoke) over(race) asyvars        ///
  ytitle("Mean birthweight (grams)")    ///
  xsize(3.9) ysize(2.2) scale(1.4)
```

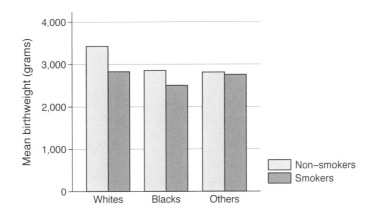

Figure 11.26: Bar graph. The `asyvars` option restructured the graph. Labels are improved.

When comparing the distribution between groups of an ordinal (rank-ordered) variable, stacked bars are efficient. In figure 11.27, the repair records of domestic and foreign cars are compared (1 is a poor and 5 a good record). In this graph, the relative bar heights should reflect the number of cars, hence the `(count)` statistic. I could have counted any variable, as long as I was sure that it had no missing values; I chose the safe way and created the help variable x. Note the use of a consistent light–dark gradient and the `order()` option to `legend()` ensuring that the legend order corresponds to the order in the bars.

```
─────────────────── gph_fig11_27.do ───────────────────
* gph_fig11_27.do

sysuse auto.dta, clear
set scheme lean2
generate x=1
graph bar (count) x                             ///
  ,                                             ///
  over(rep78) over(foreign)                     ///
  asyvars percent stack                         ///
  bar(1, fcolor(gs0))                           ///
  bar(2, fcolor(gs6))                           ///
  bar(3, fcolor(gs10))                          ///
  bar(4, fcolor(gs13))                          ///
  bar(5, fcolor(gs16))                          ///
  legend(title("Repair" "record", size(*0.8))  ///
    order(5 4 3 2 1))                           ///
  ytitle("Per cent")                            ///
  b1title("Origin")                             ///
  xsize(2.8) ysize(2.2) scale(1.4)
```

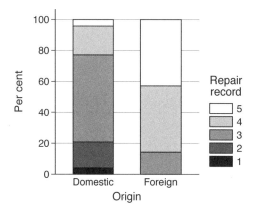

Figure 11.27: Stacked bars

Scatterplots

You have seen several scatterplots already. Markers are defined by symbol: `msymbol()`; size: `msize()`; overall color: `mcolor()`; or outline color: `mlcolor()`; and fill color: `mfcolor()`; see table 11.2 and figure 11.19.

To define a hollow circle, type

```
. twoway (scatter mpg weight, msymbol(Oh)), ...
```

A hollow circle (Oh) is transparent. You can obtain a circle with a nontransparent white fill by typing

```
. twoway (scatter mpg weight, msymbol(O) mfcolor(white)), ...
```

Figure 11.28 displays enlarged hollow triangles (Th) and small filled diamonds (d) as markers:

```
―――――――――――――― gph_fig11_28.do ――――――――――――――
* gph_fig11_28.do

sysuse auto.dta, clear
set scheme lean1

twoway                                                    ///
  (scatter mpg weight if foreign==0, msymbol(Th) msize(*1.5))  ///
  (scatter mpg weight if foreign==1, msymbol(d))             ///
  ,                                                         ///
  legend(order(1 "Domestic" 2 "Foreign"))                  ///
  xsize(3.8) ysize(2.2) scale(1.4)
```

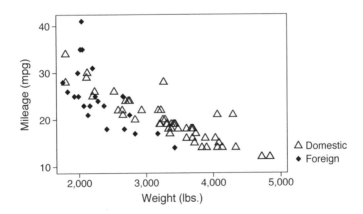

Figure 11.28: Scatterplot: Defining markers explicitly

The markers in a scatterplot may be weighted; that is, they may vary in size according to a third variable. The census.dta dataset includes demographic information for 50 U.S. states. Here we calculate urban, the degree of urbanization, and examine the relationship between urbanization and median age (medage). Each state is represented by a circle whose area is proportional to the population size (pop). I had to try a few times before I found a reasonable marker size (the msize() plot option). For information about weighting, see section 4.4.

```
                         ────────── gph_fig11_29.do ──────────
* gph_fig11_29.do

sysuse census.dta, clear
generate urban = 100*popurban/pop
label variable urban "Urbanization (per cent)"
format medage %9.0g
set scheme lean1

twoway                                                                   ///
  (scatter medage urban [fweight=pop], msymbol(Oh) msize(*0.5))          ///
  ,                                                                      ///
  yscale(range(24 35))                                                   ///
  xlabel(30(10)100)                                                      ///
  note("The marker for each state is proportional to population size")   ///
  xsize(2.9) ysize(2.2) scale(1.4)
```

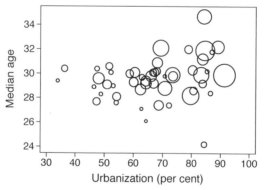

The marker for each state is proportional to population size

Figure 11.29: Weighted scatterplot

A linear regression line (see [G] **graph twoway lfit** and `lfitci`), a quadratic regression line (see [G] **graph twoway qfit** and `qfitci`), or a smoothed lowess curve (see [G] **graph twoway lowess**) can be overlaid on a scatterplot; see an example of `lfit` in figure 13.1.

Line plots

Connecting lines are used in the `twoway line` and `twoway connected` commands; for details, see [G] **graph twoway line** and [G] **graph twoway connected**. Lines are defined by `lpattern()`, `lcolor()`, and `lwidth()`; see table 11.2. Figure 11.18 shows the line patterns available.

In figure 11.30, we use the data about U.S. life expectancy to plot the life expectancy for white and black males and females. The data are in wide format, as described in section 11.2: each observation includes information on the independent variable (`year`) and the four dependent variables (`le_wmale`, `le_wfemale`, `le_bmale`, `le_bfemale`). The data are sorted by `year`; if they had not been, the result would be nonsense. The first command is rather short, but I guess it will need modifications, so I use a do-file:

```
──────────────────── gph_fig11_30.do ────────────────────
* gph_fig11_30.do

sysuse uslifeexp.dta, clear
set scheme lean2

twoway                                                      ///
  (line le_wmale le_wfemale le_bmale le_bfemale year)       ///
  ,                                                         ///
  xsize(4.4) ysize(2.2) scale(1.4)
```

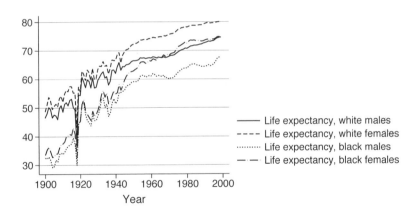

Figure 11.30: Four line plots in one plot area. Default line styles and legend.

Figure 11.30 can be improved. In figure 11.31, I chose thin lines for whites and dashed lines for males. This graph has four line plots representing four different dependent variables; in the `lpattern()` and `lwidth()` options I specified the line pattern and width for all four lines in the sequence they were mentioned in the `line` plot specification. In the `legend()` option, I chose an order corresponding to the overall sequence in the graph:

(Continued on next page)

```
──────────────── gph_fig11_31.do ────────────────
* gph_fig11_31.do

sysuse uslifeexp.dta, clear
set scheme lean2

twoway                                                ///
  (line le_wmale le_wfemale le_bmale le_bfemale year, ///
    lpattern(dash 1 dash 1) lwidth(*.8 *.8 *1.4 *1.4)) ///
  ,                                                   ///
  ytitle("Life expectancy")                           ///
  legend(order(2 "White females" 1 "White males"      ///
    4 "Black females" 3 "Black males"))               ///
  xsize(4.4) ysize(2.2) scale(1.4)
```

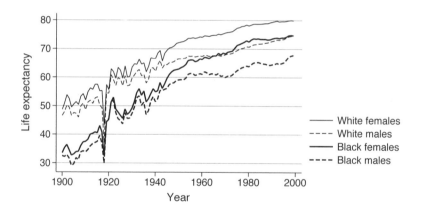

Figure 11.31: Line styles and legend text and order specified explicitly

A `twoway connected` plot is a combined line plot and scatterplot. Figure 11.32 displays the results of a study using the SF-36 questionnaire of health-related quality of life among 140 patients (obs), compared with the expected from population norm data (norm). There were a few missing values, so no scale had 140 valid observations.

```
─────────────────────── gph_fig11_32.do ───────────────────────
* gph_fig11_32.do

clear
input scale n obs sd norm
1 139 60.810 27.346 70.77
2 139 37.650 42.056 62.01
3 136 59.397 28.568 73.66
4 139 57.647 21.686 66.27
5 138 52.754 25.553 64.24
6 137 76.642 26.810 85.85
7 138 51.691 41.869 73.59
8 139 73.065 21.538 79.99
end

generate se=sd/sqrt(n)
generate ci1=obs+1.96*se
generate ci2=obs-1.96*se

label define scale 1 "PF" 2 "RP" 3 "BP" 4 "GH" 5 "VT" 6 "SF" 7 "RE" 8 "MH"
label values scale scale

set scheme lean1

twoway                                                      ///
  (connected obs scale, msymbol(O) lpattern(l))             ///
  (connected norm scale, msymbol(O) mfcolor(white) lpattern(dash))  ///
  (rcap ci1 ci2 scale)                                      ///
  ,                                                         ///
  ytitle("Mean score")                                     ///
  xtitle("SF-36 subscale")                                 ///
  xlabel(1(1)8, valuelabel noticks)                        ///
  xscale(range(0.5 8.5))                                   ///
  legend(order(2 "Expected" 1 "Observed" 3 "95% CI"))      ///
  xsize(3.9) ysize(2.2) scale(1.4)
```

(Continued on next page)

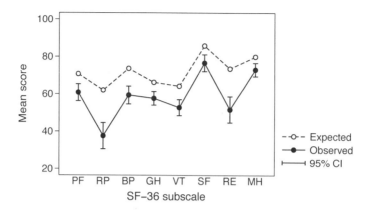

Figure 11.32: Two `connected` and one `rcap` plot

Figure 11.32 includes three plots: two `connected` and one `rcap`. In two-way plots, both axes are continuous, so you could not have a categorical variable (PF, RP, etc.) on the *x*-axis. Solution: use a numerical variable, and use value labels to indicate the meaning. This graph style is often used to present SF-36 results, although connecting lines may be illogical when displaying eight qualitatively different scales.

For the expected values, I chose a marker with a white fill; with a hollow marker (`Oh`), the connecting line would have been visible within the marker.

The *x*-axis labels could also have been defined within the `xlabel()` option:

```
. ... , xlabel(1 "PF" 2 "RP" 3 "BP" 4 "GH" 5 "VT" 6 "SF" 7 "RE" 8 "MH")
```

`xscale(range(0.5 8.5))` made the *x*-axis wider than required by the data to increase the distance between the plot symbols and the plot margin.

`rcap` is a range plot (see later this section). It does not calculate confidence intervals for you; you must provide two *y*-values and one *x*-value for each confidence interval. `rspike` (see example figure 11.33) would have plotted intervals without caps.

In figure 11.32, we entered the coordinates using the `input` command. These coordinates were obtained from the original 140 observations by the `summarize` command, but they could be generated from the original dataset by using the `statsby` command; see section 17.1. The do-file `gph_fig11_32b.do` demonstrates how this can be done; it is accessible at this book's web site.

Range plots

Figure 11.32 included a range plot (`twoway rcap`); there are other range plots; see, e.g., [G] **graph twoway rarea**, [G] **graph twoway rbar**, [G] **graph twoway rcap**, [G] **graph twoway rline**, and [G] **graph twoway rspike**. Figure 11.33 is a synthetic graph (i.e., it is created with no empirical data); the purpose is to illustrate length bias: a cross-sectional (prevalence) study may mislead you because cases with short duration (due to successful treatment or high case fatality) are underrepresented in a cross-sectional sample.

It is easy to create one or more reference lines; use xline() and yline().

```
                          ──────────── gph_fig11_33.do ────────────
* gph_fig11_33.do

clear
set obs 20                       // Create 20 empty observations
gen x=_n                         // x = observation number
gen y1=x                         // Prepare for range plot. y1=x
gen y2=x+2                        // y2=x+2
replace y2=x+8 if mod(x,2)==0    // but y2=x+8 if x is even.
set scheme lean2

twoway                                                      ///
  (rspike y1 y2 x, horizontal lwidth(*1.5))                 ///
  ,                                                         ///
  yscale(off)  ylabel(, nogrid)                             ///
  xlabel(none)  xline(14.5)  xtitle("Cross-sectional study") ///
  xsize(3.3) ysize(2.2) scale(1.4)
```

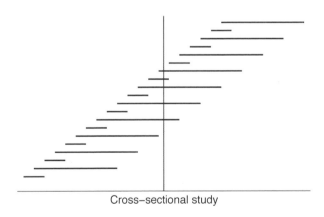

Cross–sectional study

Figure 11.33: A horizontal spike plot

Droplines

A dropline is a line going from an observation point to a baseline; see [G] **graph twoway dropline**. Figure 11.34 aims to illustrate the observation time among 14 cancer patients who were monitored during a drug trial; the observation time may end with death or censoring.

```
──────────────── gph_fig11_34.do ────────────────
* gph_fig11_34.do

sysuse cancer.dta      // Use the cancer.dta dataset accompanying Stata
keep if drug==2        // Study the 14 patients who received drug 2
sort studytime         // Sort by observation time
gen patient=_n         // and give numbers to patients

set scheme lean2

twoway                                                          ///
  (dropline studytime patient if died==1, horizontal msymbol(D))  ///
  (dropline studytime patient if died==0, horizontal msymbol(D)   ///
     mfcolor(white))                                            ///
  ,                                                             ///
  plotregion(margin(l=0 b=0))                                   ///
  ytitle("Patient number")                                     ///
  yscale(range(0 14)) ylabel(1 5 10 14, nogrid)                ///
  xtitle("Months after randomization")                        ///
  xlabel(0(6)30)                                               ///
  legend(order(1 "Death" 2 "Censoring"))                       ///
  xsize(4.4) ysize(2.2) scale(1.4)
```

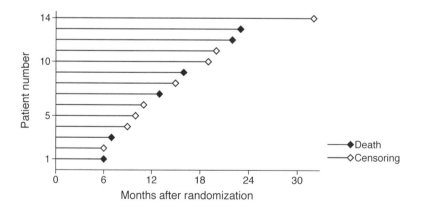

Figure 11.34: Droplines illustrating observation time in a drug trial

The baseline usually is the x- or y-axis, or rather the line with x or $y = 0$, but you can define the baseline to be 5 with the base(5) option.

The marker for censorings is a diamond with white fill, not a hollow diamond, to avoid the dropline's being visible within the marker.

Function plots

twoway function allows you to visualize mathematical functions; see [G] **graph twoway function**. Figure 11.35 is a normal distribution curve created using the normalden() function. For more information about mathematical functions, see [D] **functions**.

```
─────────────────── gph_fig11_35.do ───────────────────
* gph_fig11_35.do

set scheme lean2

twoway                                          ///
  (function y=normalden(x), range(-3.5 3.5)     ///
    droplines(-1.96 -1 0 1 1.96))               ///
  ,                                             ///
  plotregion(margin(zero))                      ///
  yscale(off) ylabel(, nogrid)                  ///
  xlabel(-3 -1.96 -1 0 1 1.96 3, format(%4.2f)) ///
  xtitle("Standard deviations from mean")       ///
  xsize(3.3) ysize(2.2) scale(1.4)
```

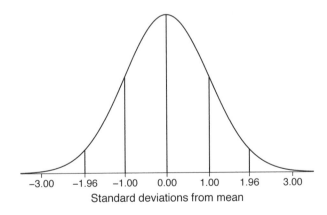

Figure 11.35: twoway function lets you plot, e.g., a normal curve.

The range() option is mandatory; it defines the *x*-axis range. droplines() is an option to function, not a separate plot command. I set the plot region margin to zero, to let the normal curve start at baseline.

Other examples:

An identity line to be overlaid in a scatterplot comparing two measurements:

```
. twoway (scatter sbp2 sbp1)(function y=x, range(sbp1))
```

A parabola:

```
. twoway (function y=x^2, range(-2 2))
```

Matrix graphs

Matrix scatterplots are useful for analysis but are rarely used for publication; see [G] **graph matrix**. They allow you to show the association between several variables in one graph.

```
————————————————————— gph_fig11_36.do —————————————————————
* gph_fig11_36.do

sysuse auto.dta, clear
set scheme lean1

graph matrix price mpg weight length, xsize(5) ysize(4)
```

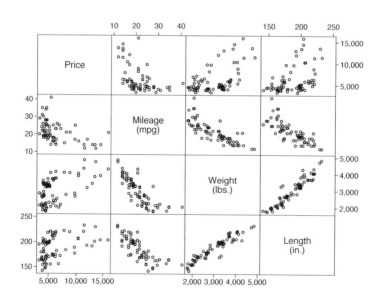

Figure 11.36: Matrix scatterplot

The upper-right cells are redundant rotated images of the lower-left cells; you can omit them by using the half option:

```
. graph matrix price mpg weight length, half
```

11.9   By-graphs and combined graphs

By-graphs

A by-graph is a graph split into two or more subgraphs (see [G] ***by_option***):

```
                          ────────── gph_fig11_37.do ──────────
* gph_fig11_37.do

sysuse auto.dta, clear
set scheme lean1

twoway (scatter mpg weight)      ///
  ,                              ///
  by(foreign, total note(""))    ///
  xsize(5) ysize(4)
```

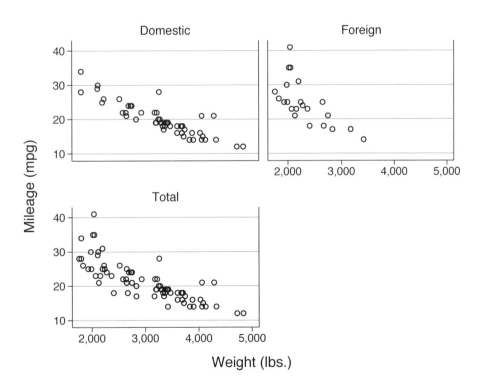

Figure 11.37: By-graph with the total option

The `total` suboption to the `by()` option displays the third graph with all observations. The `note("")` suboption removes a rather useless note ("Graphs by Car type"). You can let the graphs be stacked vertically by using the `cols()` suboption:

```
. ..., by(foreign, cols(1))
```

The rows() suboption is used similarly.

Combining graphs

You can combine several graphs with the graph combine command. In figure 11.38, three graphs are created and then combined into one figure.

```
──────────── gph_fig11_38.do ────────────
* gph_fig11_38.do

sysuse auto.dta, clear
set scheme lean1

twoway (scatter mpg weight), name(scatter, replace)

histogram mpg, frequency horizontal name(h_mpg, replace)

histogram weight, frequency name(h_weight, replace)

graph combine scatter h_mpg h_weight, xsize(5) ysize(4)
```

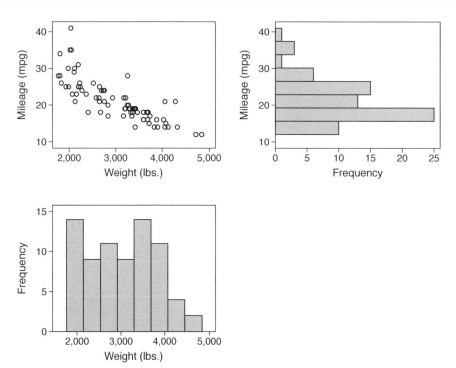

Figure 11.38: Combined graph

In figure 11.38, the individual graphs were stored as "memory graphs" by using the `name()` option; they are temporarily stored in computer memory without being written to disk. You can save them to disk with the `saving()` option:

    . ..., saving(scatter.gph, replace)

and combine them by typing

    . graph combine scatter.gph h_mpg.gph h_weight.gph

Setting `xsize()` and `ysize()` for the individual graphs before combining has no effect on the final result. There are several advanced options for combining graphs; see [G] **graph combine**.

11.10   Saving, displaying, and printing graphs

Saving a graph

You can save the current graph as a `.gph` file by typing

    . graph save lifeexp.gph [, asis replace]

The `asis` option saves a "frozen" graph, meaning that it is displayed as is, regardless of scheme settings. Without this option, you save a "live" graph: you may display it again, maybe using a different scheme or modifying its size.

You can also include a `saving()` option within the graph command:

    . ..., saving(lifeexp.gph, replace)

A saved graph may be displayed by typing

    . graph use lifeexp.gph

Save do-files rather than graph files

Rarely will you need to save graph files; instead, save a do-file for each graph with a name that tells what it does, e.g., `gph_lifeexp.do`. I recommend (Stata does not care) that you name all graph-defining do-files with a `gph` prefix, for easy identification. The do-file documents what you did, you can edit it to modify the graph, and you can modify it to create another graph. Remember to include the data or a `use` command reading the data used. This advice also applies when you have initially defined the graph command with a graph dialog.

Displaying and printing a graph

Redisplay the current graph by typing

> . graph display [, scale(1.2) ysize(3) xsize(5) scheme(lean2)]

The scale() option is useful for increasing marker and text size, for example, for a slide show. xsize() and ysize() modify the size of the graph area (arguments in inches), and scheme() lets you display a graph under a different scheme—but that sometimes fails.

Copying and printing smooth colored or gray areas sometimes give poor results, and a coarser raster pattern may be needed. This is a printer issue, not a Stata issue; in this respect modern printers are worse than older. If you encounter problems, you may experiment with selecting a coarser resolution, e.g., 300 dpi, rather than the now typical 600 or 1,200 dpi.

If you, in the future, do not want Stata's logo being printed on each graph:

> . graph set print logo off

Copying a graph to a document

To copy and paste a graph to another document, right-click the graph window, and select **Copy Graph**. Paste it to the document with **Paste Special**. In a Windows environment, the graph will be transferred as a metafile; there are two types, which you may select via the Graph Preferences menu:

> Prefs ▷ Graph Preferences ▷ Clipboard

Select Enhanced Metafile (EMF) or Windows Metafile (WMF); which one works best depends on your system and printer, so take a critical look at the results.

Submitting graphs to journals, etc.

The requirements of journals vary, but the best results are obtained by Encapsulated PostScript (.eps). The following command exports the current graph as an .eps file:

> . graph export fig3.eps, as(eps) replace

Windows metafiles (.wmf, .emf) give a reasonable quality whereas formats such as Portable Network Graphics (.png) and TIFF (.tif) give poor results.

For updated information on exporting graphs, see

> . help graph export

12 Stratified analysis

Stratified analysis and standardization are related methods for controlling confounding due to an imbalance between the groups to be compared. The general principle is stratification by the potential confounder followed by calculation of a weighted average of the information. Standardization is described in section 14.6; examples of other stratified analyses may be found in sections 12.1 and 12.2. Stratified analysis of incidence rate data is described in section 14.1.

In this chapter, I also briefly point to the regression models corresponding to the stratified analysis commands; regression analysis is demonstrated in more detail in chapter 13.

The commands in the `epitab` family perform various analyses of tabular data, including stratified analysis (Mantel–Haenszel). These commands are documented in the *Survival Analysis Manual*: [ST] **epitab**. The main `epitab` commands are as follows:

Command	Measure of association	See section	Immediate command (section 10.5)
ir	Incidence rate ratio and difference	14.1	iri
cs	Cohort studies: risk ratio and difference	12.1	csi
cc	Case–control studies: odds ratio	12.2	cci
tabodds	Odds ratio: multiple exposure levels	12.2	
mhodds	Odds ratio: continuous exposure levels	12.2	
mcc	Odds ratio: matched case–control data	12.2	mcci

> **Note!** For most `epitab` commands, the unexposed and the noncases must be coded 0 to work correctly.

12.1 Cohort data without censorings

In cohort data without censorings, the absolute risk, relative risk, and risk difference can be estimated by using `cs` (cohort study).

The `ugdp.dta` dataset describes the results from a drug trial among diabetics (University Group Diabetes Program 1970); the exposure (`exposed`) is tolbutamide, and the outcome (`case`) is death within a defined time period. The dataset is in tabular form, with pop indicating the number of subjects in each cell.

```
. webuse ugdp.dta
. numlabel, add
. list, sepby(age)
```

	age	case	exposed	pop
1.	0. <55	0	0	115
2.	0. <55	0	1	98
3.	0. <55	1	0	5
4.	0. <55	1	1	8
5.	1. 55+	0	0	69
6.	1. 55+	0	1	76
7.	1. 55+	1	0	16
8.	1. 55+	1	1	22

Here is the result of a crude analysis, one not stratified or adjusted for anything. When analyzing a tabular dataset, you must specify the cell frequencies using [fweight=*varname*] (see section 4.5):

```
. cs case exposed [fweight=pop]
```

	exposed Exposed	Unexposed	Total
Cases	30	21	51
Noncases	174	184	358
Total	204	205	409
Risk	.1470588	.102439	.1246944

	Point estimate	[95% Conf. Interval]	
Risk difference	.0446198	-.0192936	.1085332
Risk ratio	1.435574	.8510221	2.421645
Attr. frac. ex.	.3034146	-.1750577	.5870576
Attr. frac. pop	.1784792		

```
                chi2(1) =      1.87  Pr>chi2 = 0.1720
```

The crude analysis displays the risk difference (RD = 0.045; 95% CI: −0.019, 0.109) and the relative risk (RR = 1.44; 95% CI: 0.85, 2.42). The attributable risk among the exposed is 0.30; the interpretation is that among the exposed, 30% of the cases would have been avoided in the absence of the exposure. In this study, the population attributable risk has no reasonable interpretation since the exposure prevalence is determined by the proportion (50%) allocated to treatment.

Using the information in the table, the immediate command csi gives the same result:

```
. csi 30 21 174 184
```

Now let us stratify by age by typing

```
. table case exposed [fweight=pop], by(age) row col
```

Age category and case	exposed		
	0	1	Total
0. <55			
0	115	98	213
1	5	8	13
Total	120	106	226
1. 55+			
0	69	76	145
1	16	22	38
Total	85	98	183

```
. cs case exposed [fweight=pop], by(age)
```

Age category	RR	[95% Conf. Interval]		M-H Weight
0. <55	1.811321	.6112044	5.367898	2.345133
1. 55+	1.192602	.6712664	2.11883	8.568306
Crude	1.435574	.8510221	2.421645	
M-H combined	1.325555	.797907	2.202132	

Test of homogeneity (M-H)   chi2(1) =   0.447   Pr>chi2 = 0.5037

The stratification gave a modest change in the RR estimate; the difference in RRs between the young and the old may be more important (question of interaction or effect modification). However, the test of homogeneity ($Pr = 0.50$) leads us to accept a null hypothesis of a common relative risk.

It is commonplace to use logistic regression (see section 13.2) to analyze cohort data that have relative risk as the "natural" measure of association. Logistic regression, however, estimates the odds ratio, which only approximates the relative risk well under some circumstances. Binomial regression estimates relative risk directly; use binreg with the rr option:

(Continued on next page)

```
. binreg case exposed age [fweight=pop], rr
Iteration 1:    deviance =   400.6769
Iteration 2:    deviance =   296.7179
Iteration 3:    deviance =   285.7407
Iteration 4:    deviance =    285.344
Iteration 5:    deviance =   285.3425
Iteration 6:    deviance =   285.3425

Generalized linear models                 No. of obs       =        409
Optimization      : MQL Fisher scoring    Residual df      =        406
                    (IRLS EIM)            Scale parameter  =          1
Deviance          =   285.3425017         (1/df) Deviance  =    .702814
Pearson           =   405.3098098         (1/df) Pearson   =     .9983

Variance function: V(u) = u*(1-u)         [Bernoulli]
Link function    : g(u) = ln(u)           [Log]

                                          BIC              =  -2156.226
```

case	Risk Ratio	EIM Std. Err.	z	P>|z|	[95% Conf. Interval]
exposed	1.310979	.3408281	1.04	0.298	.7875904	2.182182
age	3.535708	1.081063	4.13	0.000	1.941854	6.437781

The relative risk for exposure (RR = 1.31; 95% CI: 0.79, 2.18) is close to the result of the stratified analysis with cs.

binreg with the rd option estimates risk differences:

```
. binreg case exposed age [fweight=pop], rd
Iteration 1:    deviance =   284.8929
Iteration 2:    deviance =   284.8924
Iteration 3:    deviance =   284.8924

Generalized linear models                 No. of obs       =        409
Optimization      : MQL Fisher scoring    Residual df      =        406
                    (IRLS EIM)            Scale parameter  =          1
Deviance          =   284.8924278         (1/df) Deviance  =   .7017055
Pearson           =   408.9955588         (1/df) Pearson   =   1.007378

Variance function: V(u) = u*(1-u)         [Bernoulli]
Link function    : g(u) = u               [Identity]

                                          BIC              =  -2156.676
```

case	Coef.	EIM Std. Err.	z	P>|z|	[95% Conf. Interval]
exposed	.0343372	.0278726	1.23	0.218	-.0202922	.0889666
age	.147714	.0337239	4.38	0.000	.0816164	.2138116
_cons	.041489	.0175319	2.37	0.018	.0071272	.0758508

Although it may be easier to communicate relative risks than odds ratios, analysis of binary data is usually presented as odds ratios, which have nicer mathematical properties. For an instructive discussion, see Kirkwood and Sterne (2003).

12.2 Case–control data

cc: Dichotomous exposure

In a case–control study, the odds ratio can be estimated by cc (cc for case–control). The unexposed and the noncases must be coded 0 for cc and cs (see section 12.1) to work correctly. We use the lbw1.dta dataset, studying the association between smoking and low birthweight.

In a case–control study, the exposure distribution among a group of cases is compared with the exposure distribution in the source population (the population that is the source of the cases); however, the source population is represented by a sample: the control subjects. From this design, the absolute disease risk cannot be estimated, but the relative risk can be approximated by the odds-ratio estimate. To study the association between smoking and low birthweight, we first do a crude analysis without stratification:

```
. cd C:\docs\ishr
. use lbw1.dta
(Hosmer & Lemeshow data)
. cc low smoke
```

	Exposed	Unexposed	Total	Proportion Exposed
Cases	30	29	59	0.5085
Controls	44	86	130	0.3385
Total	74	115	189	0.3915

	Point estimate	[95% Conf. Interval]		
Odds ratio	2.021944	1.029092	3.965862	(exact)
Attr. frac. ex.	.5054264	.0282693	.747848	(exact)
Attr. frac. pop	.2569965			

```
              chi2(1) =     4.92  Pr>chi2 = 0.0265
```

The crude association is OR = 2.02 (95% CI: 1.03, 3.97). The attributable risk among the exposed is 0.51, meaning that among the exposed, 51% of the cases would have been avoided in the absence of the exposure. To estimate the attributable risk in the population, the population exposure prevalence is estimated from the proportion exposed in the control group; in the absence of the exposure 26% of all cases would have been avoided, provided that the association is causal.

Using the information in the table, the immediate command cci gives the same result:

```
. cci 30 29 44 86
```

The association between smoking and birthweight might be confounded by race; a direct way to examine this is by doing a stratified analysis; the by(race) option defines the stratification variable. Below are a three-way table of the data and a stratified analysis with cc.

```
. use lbw1.dta
(Hosmer & Lemeshow data)

. table low smoke, by(race) row col stubwidth(15)
```

race and birthweight<2500g	smoked during pregnancy		
	0. No	1. Yes	Total
1. white			
0. No	40	33	73
1. Yes	4	19	23
Total	44	52	96
2. black			
0. No	11	4	15
1. Yes	5	6	11
Total	16	10	26
3. other			
0. No	35	7	42
1. Yes	20	5	25
Total	55	12	67

```
. cc low smoke, by(race)
```

race	OR	[95% Conf. Interval]		M-H Weight	
1. white	5.757576	1.657574	25.1388	1.375	(exact)
2. black	3.3	.4865385	23.45437	.7692308	(exact)
3. other	1.25	.273495	5.278229	2.089552	(exact)
Crude	2.021944	1.029092	3.965864		(exact)
M-H combined	3.086381	1.49074	6.389949		

```
Test of homogeneity (M-H)      chi2(2) =      3.03  Pr>chi2 = 0.2197
                    Test that combined OR = 1:
                              Mantel-Haenszel chi2(1) =       9.41
                                            Pr>chi2 =      0.0022
```

Without stratification, the odds ratio (crude OR) is 2.02 (95% CI: 1.03, 3.97), whereas the Mantel–Haenszel adjusted odds ratio is 3.09 (95% CI: 1.49, 6.39). The odds ratios for the three strata are rather different, but the confidence intervals are wide, and the test of homogeneity (Pr = 0.22) does not reject the hypothesis that they represent a common odds ratio (question of interaction or effect modification).

You can stratify only by one variable, but the following egen command lets you generate a new variable (htrace) combining the categories of two variables (ht and race). The label option generates value labels for the new variable.

```
. egen htrace=group(ht race), label
. cc low smoke, by(htrace)
```

group(ht race)	OR	[95% Conf. Interval]		M-H Weight	
0. No 1. white	5.346774	1.505951	23.66822	1.362637	(exact)
0. No 2. black	3.125	.3992806	25.30971	.6956522	(exact)
0. No 3. other	1.428571	.3072007	6.120892	1.888889	(exact)
1. Yes 1. white	.	0	.	0	(exact)
1. Yes 2. black	.	0	.	0	(exact)
1. Yes 3. other	.	.	.	0	(exact)
Crude	2.021944	1.029092	3.965864		(exact)
M-H combined	3.265972	1.553342	6.866853		

```
Test of homogeneity (B-D)      chi2(5) =      2.88  Pr>chi2 = 0.7192

               Test that combined OR = 1:
                       Mantel-Haenszel chi2(1) =       9.83
                                       Pr>chi2 =     0.0017
```

The example illustrates that there are limits to stratification: three strata (those with hypertension) become so thin that they contribute no information. In such cases, a regression model is preferable.

The regression model corresponding to stratified analysis of case–control data is logistic regression, which also estimates odds ratios; see section 13.2.

```
. xi: logistic low smoke ht i.race
i.race              _Irace_1-3        (naturally coded; _Irace_1 omitted)

Logistic regression                        Number of obs   =        189
                                           LR chi2(4)      =      18.32
                                           Prob > chi2     =     0.0011
Log likelihood = -108.17506               Pseudo R2       =     0.0781
```

low	Odds Ratio	Std. Err.	z	P>|z|	[95% Conf. Interval]	
smoke	3.094613	1.155266	3.03	0.002	1.488812	6.432395
ht	3.252896	2.028429	1.89	0.059	.9582548	11.04229
_Irace_2	2.803324	1.393426	2.07	0.038	1.058213	7.426313
_Irace_3	3.06541	1.240313	2.77	0.006	1.387008	6.774827

tabodds: Multiple exposure levels

To study the effect of multiple exposure levels in a case–control study, use tabodds; see [ST] **epitab**. The data are from the much-cited Ille-et-Villaine study of risk factors for esophageal cancer (Breslow and Day 1980). The alcohol consumption (grams/day) is recorded in four levels. freq is the number of cases or controls in each exposure category, hence [fweight=freq] in the tabodds command. The or option displays odds ratios; without it, tabodds displays absolute odds, which in a case–control study reflect design decisions more than anything else:

```
. webuse bdesop.dta, clear
. numlabel, add
. tabodds case alcohol [fweight=freq], or
```

alcohol	Odds Ratio	chi2	P>chi2	[95% Conf. Interval]	
1. 0-39	1.000000	.	.	.	.
2. 40-79	3.565271	32.70	0.0000	2.237981	5.679744
3. 80-119	7.802616	75.03	0.0000	4.497054	13.537932
4. 120+	27.225705	160.41	0.0000	12.507808	59.262107

```
Test of homogeneity (equal odds): chi2(3)  =    158.79
                                   Pr>chi2  =    0.0000

Score test for trend of odds:      chi2(1)  =    152.97
                                   Pr>chi2  =    0.0000
```

The tests of homogeneity and trend in `tabodds` refer to the dose–response association, whereas in most other commands, they refer to differences between strata (effect modification, interaction).

To adjust by stratification for another exposure, use the `adjust()` option:

```
. tabodds case alcohol [fweight=freq], adjust(tobacco)
Mantel-Haenszel odds ratios adjusted for tobacco
```

alcohol	Odds Ratio	chi2	P>chi2	[95% Conf. Interval]	
1. 0-39	1.000000	.	.	.	.
2. 40-79	3.261178	28.53	0.0000	2.059764	5.163349
3. 80-119	6.771638	62.54	0.0000	3.908113	11.733306
4. 120+	19.919526	123.93	0.0000	9.443830	42.015528

```
Score test for trend of odds: chi2(1)  =   135.04
                              Pr>chi2  =   0.0000
```

The corresponding logistic regression analysis follows:

```
. xi: logistic case i.alcohol i.tobacco [fweight=freq]
i.alcohol          _Ialcohol_1-4      (naturally coded; _Ialcohol_1 omitted)
i.tobacco          _Itobacco_1-4      (naturally coded; _Itobacco_1 omitted)

Logistic regression                      Number of obs   =        975
                                         LR chi2(6)      =     159.13
                                         Prob > chi2     =     0.0000
Log likelihood =     -415.18            Pseudo R2       =     0.1608
```

case	Odds Ratio	Std. Err.	z	P>|z|	[95% Conf. Interval]	
_Ialcohol_2	3.402691	.7976312	5.22	0.000	2.149269	5.387091
_Ialcohol_3	7.373851	1.949248	7.56	0.000	4.392206	12.37958
_Ialcohol_4	24.04584	7.872427	9.71	0.000	12.65794	45.67904
_Itobacco_2	1.471323	.3113935	1.82	0.068	.9717577	2.227706
_Itobacco_3	1.529773	.3919808	1.66	0.097	.9258051	2.527751
_Itobacco_4	2.685142	.7770595	3.41	0.001	1.522776	4.734765

The odds-ratio estimate for _Ialcohol_2 corresponds to tabodds' odds ratio for the category 40–79 g/day, the first category (0–39) being the reference. The estimates are not identical because of different estimation principles, but the general pattern remains.

mhodds: Continuous exposure levels

mhodds performs simple and stratified analysis for case–control data where the exposure variable is on a continuous scale. The odds ratio is interpreted as the odds ratio per unit increase in the exposure.

Although the exposure (alcohol) is not recorded as a continuous variable in the esophagus cancer data, but as four exposure levels (coded 1–4), we will use these data for comparison with tabodds:

```
. webuse bdesop.dta, clear
. mhodds case alcohol [fweight=freq]
Score test for trend of odds with alcohol
(The Odds Ratio estimate is an approximation to the odds ratio
for a one unit increase in alcohol)
```

Odds Ratio	chi2(1)	P>chi2	[95% Conf. Interval]	
2.951639	152.97	0.0000	2.486415	3.503910

The interpretation is that when using group 1 (0–39 g/day) as the reference category, the odds ratio for group 2 is 2.95, for group 3 it is $2.95^2 = 8.70$, and for group 4 it is $2.95^3 = 25.7$. You could compare these results with those found by tabodds and conclude that the results from the two analyses are similar. The score test for trend in tabodds gave exactly the same chi-squared value; that is no accident, as it is the same analysis.

You can make a stratified analysis (the by() option) and see the odds ratios for the alcohol–cancer association in each stratum, and the Mantel–Haenszel, weighted common estimate:

(Continued on next page)

```
. numlabel, add
. mhodds case alcohol [fweight=freq], by(tobacco)
```

Score test for trend of odds with alcohol
by tobacco

(The Odds Ratio estimate is an approximation to the odds ratio
for a one unit increase in alcohol)

tobacco	Odds Ratio	chi2(1)	P>chi2	[95% Conf. Interval]	
1. 0-9	3.906025	88.00	0.0000	2.93832	5.19244
2. 10-19	2.359218	28.11	0.0000	1.71781	3.24012
3. 20-29	2.168829	12.00	0.0005	1.39956	3.36093
4. 30+	2.323704	15.36	0.0001	1.52429	3.54237

Mantel-Haenszel estimate controlling for tobacco

Odds Ratio	chi2(1)	P>chi2	[95% Conf. Interval]	
2.802198	135.04	0.0000	2.355175	3.334069

Test of homogeneity of ORs (approx): chi2(3) =   8.43
                                     Pr>chi2 = 0.0379

The adjusted odds ratio does not differ much from the crude estimate. Finally, you can see the test of homogeneity of odds ratios across strata; $p = 0.04$ (and this time it really is a test of homogeneity). You may conclude that there is a significant interaction (or effect-measure modification): the level of tobacco use modifies the effect of alcohol when using the odds-ratio as the effect measure, and you should probably avoid reporting a single odds-ratio estimate. The finding that those with the lowest exposure to a competing risk factor have the highest *relative* risk (or odds ratio) is common: the denominator in the relative-risk calculation is small. Looking at absolute risks might be informative, but usually case–control designs do not allow that.

You might also stratify for tobacco by including it as a third variable in the *varlist*. The result is the same, but with this syntax the individual strata and the test of homogeneity are not displayed.

```
. mhodds case alcohol tobacco [fweight=freq]
```

Score test for trend of odds with alcohol
controlling for tobacco

(The Odds Ratio estimate is an approximation to the odds ratio
for a one unit increase in alcohol)

Odds Ratio	chi2(1)	P>chi2	[95% Conf. Interval]	
2.802198	135.04	0.0000	2.355175	3.334069

The corresponding logistic regression analysis is

```
. xi: logistic case alcohol i.tobacco [fweight=freq]
i.tobacco          _Itobacco_1-4     (naturally coded; _Itobacco_1 omitted)
```

```
Logistic regression                          Number of obs   =        975
                                             LR chi2(4)      =     157.61
                                             Prob > chi2     =     0.0000
Log likelihood =   -415.937                  Pseudo R2       =     0.1593
```

case	Odds Ratio	Std. Err.	z	P>|z|	[95% Conf. Interval]	
alcohol	2.751469	.2610628	10.67	0.000	2.284555	3.313811
_Itobacco_2	1.461981	.3092472	1.80	0.073	.9658066	2.213059
_Itobacco_3	1.572017	.401791	1.77	0.077	.9525744	2.594271
_Itobacco_4	2.711107	.7831288	3.45	0.001	1.539108	4.775559

The odds ratio for alcohol does not differ much from what we found with mhodds. Whereas mhodds with the by() option made the effect modification quite visible, we might easily miss it with a regression analysis.

mhodds is more flexible than cc; e.g., it allows more than one stratification variable. The confidence intervals differ a bit due to different estimation principles:

```
. cd C:\docs\ishr
```

```
. use lbw1.dta, clear
(Hosmer & Lemeshow data)
```

```
. mhodds low smoke, by(ht race)
Maximum likelihood estimate of the odds ratio
Comparing smoke==1 vs. smoke==0
by ht race
note: only 5 of the 6 strata formed in this analysis contribute
      information about the effect of the explanatory variable
```

ht	race	Odds Ratio	chi2(1)	P>chi2	[95% Conf. Interval]	
0. No	1. white	5.346774	8.62	0.0033	1.52411	18.75719
0. No	2. black	3.125000	1.60	0.2056	0.48575	20.10425
0. No	3. other	1.428571	0.29	0.5889	0.38923	5.24326
1. Yes	1. white	.	0.67	0.4142	.	.
1. Yes	2. black	.	0.50	0.4795	.	.
1. Yes	3. other	.	.	.	.	.

```
    Mantel-Haenszel estimate controlling for ht and race
```

Odds Ratio	chi2(1)	P>chi2	[95% Conf. Interval]	
3.265972	9.83	0.0017	1.491248	7.152783

```
Test of homogeneity of ORs (approx): chi2(4)  =     2.61
                                     Pr>chi2  =   0.6254
```

mcc: Analyzing matched case–control data

Matching in case–control studies may be used to attempt to control for confounding and to improve study efficiency. However, matched case–control studies require special treatment to obtain valid results: the matched sets (a case and its matched controls) must be kept together in the analysis, using a set identifier as a stratification variable.

The lowbirth.dta dataset is a modification of the lbw.dta dataset; we now have 56 case–control pairs matched on age (a 1:1 match) (Hosmer and Lemeshow 2000). The key variables are pairid (each case and her matching controls constitute a set), low (1: cases; 0: controls), and smoke (1: smokers, 0: nonsmokers):

```
. webuse lowbirth.dta, clear
(Applied Logistic Regression, Hosmer & Lemeshow)

. keep pairid low smoke

. list in 1/6, sepby(pairid)
```

	pairid	low	smoke
1.	1	0	0
2.	1	1	1
3.	2	0	0
4.	2	1	0
5.	3	0	0
6.	3	1	0

This dataset is in long format, but the mcc command requires a wide format with the information on a case and her matching control in the same observation. We use reshape (see section 9.6):

```
. reshape wide smoke, i(pairid) j(low)
(note: j = 0 1)
```

Data	long	->	wide
Number of obs.	112	->	56
Number of variables	3	->	3
j variable (2 values)	low	->	(dropped)
xij variables:			
	smoke	->	smoke0 smoke1

```
. list in 1/3
```

	pairid	smoke0	smoke1
1.	1	0	1
2.	2	0	0
3.	3	0	0

Each observation now constitutes a set, with smoke0 containing information on exposure of the control and smoke1 containing the exposure of the case. To perform the analysis, type

```
. mcc smoke1 smoke0

                  | Controls
Cases             | Exposed   Unexposed        Total
------------------+--------------------------------------
        Exposed   |    8         22              30
      Unexposed   |    8         18              26
------------------+--------------------------------------
          Total   |   16         40              56

McNemar's chi2(1) =      6.53    Prob > chi2 = 0.0106
Exact McNemar significance probability      = 0.0161

Proportion with factor
        Cases       .5357143
        Controls    .2857143           [95% Conf. Interval]
                    ----------
        difference       .25      .0519726    .4480274
        ratio          1.875      1.148685    3.060565
        rel. diff.       .35      .1336258    .5663742

        odds ratio      2.75      1.179154    7.143667    (exact)
```

mcc performs McNemar's test for matched pairs and displays several estimates, of which the odds ratio is the most interesting (OR = 2.75; 95% CI: 1.18, 7.14).

Using the information in the table, the immediate command mcci gives the same result:

```
. mcci 8 22 8 18
```

mcc simply performed an analysis stratifying by pairid. In the table above, we see $22 + 8$ informative pairs, while the $8 + 18$ pairs with the same exposure for cases and controls provide no information; the odds-ratio estimate is $22/8 = 2.75$. We can obtain almost the same estimate with cc without a reshape. The confidence intervals differ somewhat; mcc's exact confidence interval is the most accurate:

```
. webuse lowbirth.dta, clear
(Applied Logistic Regression, Hosmer & Lemeshow)

. cc low smoke, by(pairid)

Case-control pai |      OR     [95% Conf. Interval]    M-H Weight
-----------------+---------------------------------------------------
              1  |      .          0          .           0  (exact)
              2  |      .          .          .           0  (exact)
                     (output omitted )
             55  |      .          0          .           0  (exact)
             56  |      .          0          .           0  (exact)
-----------------+---------------------------------------------------
         Crude   |  2.884615   1.232782   6.820112          (exact)
    M-H combined |     2.75    1.224347   6.176763
-----------------+---------------------------------------------------

            Test that combined OR = 1:
                      Mantel-Haenszel chi2(1) =       6.53
                                      Pr>chi2 =     0.0106
```

cc produced quite a long and not very informative table with 56 strata; you can obtain the same without the table—and get some more information—by using mhodds:

. mhodds low smoke pairid

```
Mantel-Haenszel estimate of the odds ratio
Comparing smoke==1 vs. smoke==0, controlling for pairid

note: only 30 of the 56 strata formed in this analysis contribute
      information about the effect of the explanatory variable
```

Odds Ratio	chi2(1)	P>chi2	[95% Conf. Interval]	
2.750000	6.53	0.0106	1.224347	6.176763

The appropriate regression model for matched case–control data is conditional logistic regression. Whereas we analyzed 1:1 matched data above, clogit analyzes any matching ratio, including varying number of controls, and it allows controlling for more confounders; see section 13.4:

. clogit low smoke, group(pairid) or

```
Iteration 0:   log likelihood = -35.425931
Iteration 1:   log likelihood = -35.419283
Iteration 2:   log likelihood = -35.419282
```

```
Conditional (fixed-effects) logistic regression    Number of obs   =        112
                                                   LR chi2(1)      =       6.79
                                                   Prob > chi2     =     0.0091
Log likelihood = -35.419282                        Pseudo R2       =     0.0875
```

low	Odds Ratio	Std. Err.	z	P>|z|	[95% Conf. Interval]	
smoke	2.75	1.135369	2.45	0.014	1.224347	6.176763

13   Regression analysis

This chapter describes the fundamentals of linear regression and logistic regression. There are, however, many other regression models available in Stata. Chapter 14 discusses Poisson regression and Cox regression; the general principles apply to them, too.

Performing regression analysis with Stata is easy. Defining regression models that make sense and interpreting the results is more complex. Especially consider the following:

- If you study a causal hypothesis, make sure that your model is meaningful. Do not include independent variables that may represent steps in the causal pathway; they may create more confounding than it prevents. Automatic selection procedures are available in Stata (see [R] **stepwise**), but they may seduce the user into not thinking. I will therefore not describe them.

- If your hypothesis is noncausal and you look only for predictors, logical requirements are more relaxed, but at least the time relations should be meaningful.

- Take care with closely associated independent variables, such as education and social class. Including both may obscure more information than it illuminates.

Kirkwood and Sterne (2003) give good advice on several general issues in regression modeling.

13.1   Linear regression

A linear regression expresses the dependency of one variable (the response, outcome, or dependent variable) on one or more other variables (predictors, regressors, or independent variables). For extensive documentation, see [R] **regress**.

(Continued on next page)

We use the `auto.dta` dataset: with `mpg` (mileage) as the dependent variable and `weight` as a predictor, the `regress` command gives the following output:

```
. sysuse auto.dta, clear
(1978 Automobile Data)

. regress mpg weight

      Source |       SS       df       MS              Number of obs =      74
-------------+------------------------------           F(  1,    72) =  134.62
       Model | 1591.9902        1  1591.9902           Prob > F      =  0.0000
    Residual | 851.469256      72 11.8259619           R-squared     =  0.6515
-------------+------------------------------           Adj R-squared =  0.6467
       Total | 2443.45946      73 33.4720474           Root MSE      =  3.4389

------------------------------------------------------------------------------
         mpg |      Coef.   Std. Err.      t    P>|t|     [95% Conf. Interval]
-------------+----------------------------------------------------------------
      weight |  -.0060087   .0005179   -11.60   0.000    -.0070411   -.0049763
       _cons |   39.44028   1.614003    24.44   0.000     36.22283    42.65774
------------------------------------------------------------------------------
```

The last part of the output with the regression coefficients is the most important. It can be translated to

Predicted `mpg` = 39.44 miles/gallon − 0.006 × weight

A difference in weight of 1,000 lb. corresponds to a predicted difference in mileage of −6 miles per gallon; the 95% confidence interval is (−7, −5) miles per gallon. The result is highly significant ($t = -11.6$; Pr < 0.001). `_cons` is the constant or intercept, i.e., the predicted outcome when all predictors are 0. Here it is the predicted mileage (39.4 miles per gallon) for a car with a weight of 0 lb. Extrapolations outside the observed ranges of the predictors can lead to nonsense, but the intercept informs you about the general level of the outcome.

The R-squared statistic (R^2) of 0.65 is the *coefficient of determination* and is interpreted as the proportion of the variation in mileage that is "explained" by the cars' weights. In figure 13.1, a scatterplot with a regression line illustrates the association. Here we show the minimum graph command; you can find a do-file with the full command (`gph_fig13_1.do`) at this book's web site.

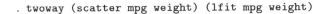

```
. twoway (scatter mpg weight) (lfit mpg weight)
```

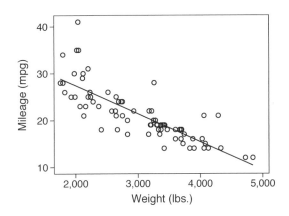

Figure 13.1: Scatterplot with a regression line

Regression diagnostics

The main requirements for a linear regression analysis to be valid are as follows:

- The association should be linear.
- The residuals (observed–predicted mpg) should be normally distributed.
- The variation of the residuals should be independent of the level of mpg (homoskedasticity).

You can read more in [R] **regress postestimation**.

Looking at the scatterplot in figure 13.1, the association is obvious, but a straight line may not be the best description. The residuals can be amended to the dataset with the predict command right after the regression analysis, and the distribution can be examined in a histogram. predict (see [R] **predict**) is a postestimation command; from the regression coefficients, it creates a new variable: the predicted mpg for each observation. To make sure that the prediction applies only to the observations included in the regression analyses, use e(sample):

(*Continued on next page*)

```
. predict pmpg if e(sample)
. label variable pmpg "Predicted mpg"
. generate rmpg = mpg - pmpg
. label variable rmpg "Residual (mpg)"
. histogram rmpg, frequency normal
```

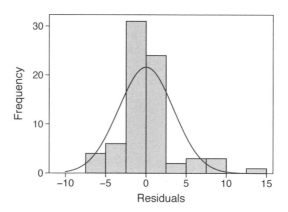

Figure 13.2: Histogram of residuals; normal curve overlaid

You could also obtain the residual directly with the following:

```
. predict rmpg if e(sample), residual
```

The residual distribution in figure 13.2 does not seem to be normal; this supposition can be tested formally with the `swilk` command:

```
. swilk rmpg
```

	Shapiro-Wilk W test for normal data				
Variable	Obs	W	V	z	Prob>z
rmpg	74	0.89593	6.702	4.150	0.00002

The Shapiro–Wilk test leads us to reject the hypothesis that the residuals are from a normal distribution. However, with large datasets (this is not one), even unimportant departures from normality become significant, and visual inspection is the most important tool.

The requirement that the residual variation is constant across the predicted levels (homoskedasticity) can be examined by `rvfplot` (residual versus fitted); this command should also be issued after a regression analysis:

```
. rvfplot, yline(0)
```

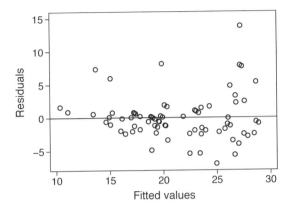

Figure 13.3: Residual-versus-fitted plot

The residual variation seems to increase with increasing predicted values of mpg, and the requirement of homoskedasticity is not fulfilled.

In conclusion, this was a case where the requirements for linear regression were not fulfilled, and although we do not doubt that there is a strong association between the cars' weight and mileage, the linear regression model is probably not the best description. One possible solution is a transformation of the dependent variable. In section 10.4, the output from gladder led to the suggestion to make an inverse transformation of mpg; I chose to express it as gallons per 100 miles:

```
. generate gp100m = 100/mpg
. label variable gp100m "Gallons per 100 miles"
```

Now we could run a regression with gp100m as the dependent variable and look at the results. We could make a scatterplot like figure 13.1 and diagnostic plots like figures 13.2 and 13.3, and evaluate the results. Then we could compare the R^2 values from the two analyses.

Cox (2004) surveys a whole family of regression diagnostic graphs; you can find it by typing

```
. findit modeldiag
```

Regression analysis with several independent variables

We will now turn to the lbw1.dta dataset on predictors of low birthweight used in chapter 10. describe tells us about the dataset:

```
. cd C:\docs\ishr

. use lbw1.dta, clear
(Hosmer & Lemeshow data)

. describe

Contains data from C:\docs\ishr\lbw1.dta
  obs:            189                          Hosmer & Lemeshow data
  vars:            11                          2 Apr 2005 21:10
  size:         3,402 (99.9% of memory free)
```

variable name	storage type	display format	value label	variable label
id	int	%8.0g		identification code
low	byte	%8.0g	yesno	birthweight<2500g
age	byte	%8.0g		age of mother
lwt	int	%8.0g		weight at last menstrual period
race	byte	%8.0g	race	race
smoke	byte	%8.0g	yesno	smoked during pregnancy
ptl	byte	%8.0g		premature labor history (count)
ht	byte	%8.0g	yesno	has history of hypertension
ui	byte	%8.0g	yesno	presence, uterine irritability
ftv	byte	%8.0g		number of visits to physician during 1st trimester
bwt	int	%8.0g		birthweight (grams)

```
Sorted by:
```

We hypothesize that maternal age (age), prepregnancy weight (lwt), and smoking (smoke) influence birthweight. Actually, smoking is the factor of interest, but smoking may be associated with maternal age and weight, and without controlling for these factors, we might misinterpret the causal effect of smoking (a confounding problem). age and lwt are continuous variables, but smoke is dichotomous, and we must know how it is coded to interpret the results. Fortunately, we used numlabel to add codes to the value labels:

```
. tab1 smoke

-> tabulation of smoke
```

smoked during pregnancy	Freq.	Percent	Cum.
0. No	115	60.85	60.85
1. Yes	74	39.15	100.00
Total	189	100.00	

```
. regress bwt age lwt smoke
```

Source	SS	df	MS
Model	7000336.31	3	2333445.44
Residual	92914962.3	185	502243.039
Total	99915298.6	188	531464.354

```
Number of obs =      189
F(  3,   185) =     4.65
Prob > F      =   0.0037
R-squared     =   0.0701
Adj R-squared =   0.0550
Root MSE      =   708.69
```

bwt	Coef.	Std. Err.	t	P>|t|	[95% Conf. Interval]	
age	7.040796	9.923378	0.71	0.479	-12.53674	26.61833
lwt	4.020133	1.719721	2.34	0.020	.6273465	7.412919
smoke	-268.146	105.7908	-2.53	0.012	-476.8575	-59.43464
_cons	2363.765	300.6933	7.86	0.000	1770.537	2956.994

From the small $R^2 = 0.07$, we can see that these predictors explain only little of the variation in birthweight. The association with age is insignificant, but there is a tendency toward increased birthweight with increasing maternal age (7 g per year). There is a significant association with the mother's prepregnancy weight (lwt) of 4 g per lb. The coefficient for smoke is -268 g (95% CI: -477, -59), meaning that when controlling for maternal age and prepregnancy weight, smokers had babies that were on average 268 g lighter than those of nonsmokers.

With three independent variables, the relationship cannot be displayed graphically, but you can still calculate the residuals (predict) and use rvfplot to examine them.

Right after issuing the regression command, you can estimate the expected birthweight for, e.g., a newborn whose mother is 30 years old, weighs 120 lb., and smokes; see [R] **lincom**:

```
. lincom 30*age + 120*lwt + smoke + _cons
( 1)   30 age + 120 lwt + smoke + _cons = 0
```

bwt	Coef.	Std. Err.	t	P>|t|	[95% Conf. Interval]	
(1)	2789.259	110.5992	25.22	0.000	2571.061	3007.457

The result from lincom depends on the preceding regression command. Here

```
. lincom 30*age + _cons
```

is the same as

```
. lincom 30*age + 0*lwt + 0*smoke + _cons
```

so we get the predicted birthweight for 30-year-old nonsmoking mothers with a prepregnancy weight of 0!

The `adjust` command can be used for similar purposes; see [R] **adjust**.

```
. adjust age=30 lwt=120, by(smoke) se ci
```

```
     Dependent variable: bwt     Command: regress
Covariates set to value: age = 30, lwt = 120
```

smoked during pregnancy	xb	stdp	lb	ub
0. No	3057.41	(97.0107)	[2866.02	3248.79]
1. Yes	2789.26	(110.599)	[2571.06	3007.46]

```
Key:  xb     =  Linear Prediction
      stdp   =  Standard Error
      [lb , ub] =  [95% Confidence Interval]
```

If you had not specified values for `age` and `lwt`, they would be set to their mean values.

Working with categorical predictors: The xi: prefix

We wish to include `race` in the list of predictors. The purpose may be to control for confounding by race when we are estimating the independent effect of smoking, or we may be interested in the effect of race itself on birthweight. The coding of `race` is

```
. tab1 race
-> tabulation of race
```

race	Freq.	Percent	Cum.
1. white	96	50.79	50.79
2. black	26	13.76	64.55
3. other	67	35.45	100.00
Total	189	100.00	

`race` is on a nominal scale; the codes themselves (1, 2, 3) are just codes, and there is no point in using them as values in any analysis. We want to contrast the birthweight among blacks and among others with that of white mothers. To do this, we need to construct *dummy* or indicator variables, i.e., dichotomous variables that may be used. One way to do this is to let `tab1` generate them. (`quietly` suppresses the display of the table, and `generate()` creates a new dichotomous variable for each value of `race`. For the `groups` command, see section 10.3.)

```
. quietly tab1 race, generate(race)

. groups race*
```

race	race1	race2	race3	Freq.	Percent
1. white	1	0	0	96	50.79
2. black	0	1	0	26	13.76
3. other	0	0	1	67	35.45

Now we can run the regression with the new dummy variables (race? means all variables starting with race and having exactly one more character):

```
. regress bwt smoke race?
```

Source	SS	df	MS		Number of obs =	189
					F(3, 185) =	8.69
Model	12346897.6	3	4115632.54		Prob > F =	0.0000
Residual	87568400.9	185	473342.708		R-squared =	0.1236
					Adj R-squared =	0.1094
Total	99915298.6	188	531464.354		Root MSE =	688

bwt	Coef.	Std. Err.	t	P>|t|	[95% Conf. Interval]	
smoke	-428.0254	109.0033	-3.93	0.000	-643.0746	-212.9761
race1	450.54	153.066	2.94	0.004	148.5607	752.5194
race2	(dropped)					
race3	-3.641269	160.537	-0.02	0.982	-320.3599	313.0773
_cons	2884.317	141.291	20.41	0.000	2605.569	3163.066

Stata dropped race2 from the analysis because it contributed no information beyond race1 and race3; the information in a variable with three categories can be expressed with two dummy variables. The effect was that race2 (the blacks) became the reference group with which the birthweight of whites and others were compared. However, we want the whites to be the reference group—one good reason is that it is the largest group—so we omit this variable (race1) from the command

```
. regress bwt smoke race2 race3
```

Source	SS	df	MS		Number of obs =	189
					F(3, 185) =	8.69
Model	12346897.6	3	4115632.54		Prob > F =	0.0000
Residual	87568400.9	185	473342.708		R-squared =	0.1236
					Adj R-squared =	0.1094
Total	99915298.6	188	531464.354		Root MSE =	688

bwt	Coef.	Std. Err.	t	P>|t|	[95% Conf. Interval]	
smoke	-428.0254	109.0033	-3.93	0.000	-643.0746	-212.9761
race2	-450.54	153.066	-2.94	0.004	-752.5194	-148.5607
race3	-454.1813	116.436	-3.90	0.000	-683.8944	-224.4683
_cons	3334.858	91.74301	36.35	0.000	3153.86	3515.855

The average birthweight among blacks (race2) was 451 g lower than among whites, and birthweight among others (race3) 454 g lower than among whites, when controlling for maternal smoking.

Stata has an elegant way to construct the dummy variables, the xi: prefix (see [R] **xi**):

```
. xi: regress bwt i.smoke i.race
i.smoke          _Ismoke_0-1         (naturally coded; _Ismoke_0 omitted)
i.race           _Irace_1-3          (naturally coded; _Irace_1 omitted)

      Source |       SS       df       MS              Number of obs =     189
-------------+------------------------------           F(  3,   185) =    8.69
       Model | 12346897.6        3  4115632.54         Prob > F      =  0.0000
    Residual | 87568400.9      185  473342.708         R-squared     =  0.1236
-------------+------------------------------           Adj R-squared =  0.1094
       Total | 99915298.6      188  531464.354         Root MSE      =     688

-------------+----------------------------------------------------------------
         bwt |      Coef.   Std. Err.      t    P>|t|     [95% Conf. Interval]
-------------+----------------------------------------------------------------
   _Ismoke_1 |  -428.0254   109.0033    -3.93   0.000    -643.0746   -212.9761
    _Irace_2 |   -450.54    153.066     -2.94   0.004    -752.5194   -148.5607
    _Irace_3 |  -454.1813   116.436     -3.90   0.000    -683.8944   -224.4683
       _cons |  3334.858   91.74301     36.35   0.000     3153.86    3515.855
```

This result is identical to that of the preceding analysis. xi: created three new dichotomous variables (coded 0/1), _Ismoke_1, _Irace_2, and _Irace_3; see the output from describe:

```
. describe
(output omitted)

              storage  display      value
variable name   type   format       label     variable label
----------------------------------------------------------------------
id              int    %8.0g                   identification code
(output omitted)
_Ismoke_1       byte   %8.0g                   smoke==1
_Irace_2        byte   %8.0g                   race==2
_Irace_3        byte   %8.0g                   race==3
----------------------------------------------------------------------
Sorted by:
```

By default, the first (lowest) category will be omitted in the construction of dummy variables; here it meant that nonsmokers (smoke = 0) and whites (race = 1) became the reference groups. If you wanted blacks (race = 2) to be the reference group, you could do that by assigning a "characteristic" to race (see [R] **xi**):

```
. char race[omit] 2
```

If you save the dataset, the dummy variables and characteristics are saved with it.

In the above regression, you see separate significance tests for _Irace2 (blacks versus whites) and _Irace3 (others versus whites). You might, however, want to test the overall difference between races, so you could use test and testparm (see [R] **test**). Like lincom, the command must be run right after the estimation command. Here we find a significant overall difference in birthweight between races:

```
. quietly xi: regress bwt i.smoke i.race
. testparm _Irace*
 ( 1)  _Irace_2 = 0
 ( 2)  _Irace_3 = 0
       F(  2,   185) =    9.24
             Prob > F =    0.0001
```

Interactions in regression analysis

The effect of smoking on birthweight might be different among whites, blacks, and others. This phenomenon is called *interaction* or *effect modification* and can be studied by comparing the observed and predicted values of the dependent variable after running a regression analysis (the analysis shown above):

```
. quietly xi: regress bwt i.smoke i.race
. predict pbwt if e(sample)
(option xb assumed; fitted values)
. gen resid = bwt - pbwt
. table smoke, by(race) c(mean bwt mean pbwt mean resid) format(%8.0f)
> stubw(18)
```

race and smoked during pregnancy		mean(bwt)	mean(pbwt)	mean(resid)
1. white				
	0. No	3429	3335	94
	1. Yes	2827	2907	-79
2. black				
	0. No	2854	2884	-30
	1. Yes	2504	2456	48
3. other				
	0. No	2814	2881	-66
	1. Yes	2757	2453	305

For the observed values (bwt), you see a large difference between smoking and nonsmoking white women (602 g), whereas the difference is small (57 g) for women of "other" race. For the predicted values (pbwt), you see the same difference for all races (428 g). The regression model used assumes the same effect across races, and the discrepancies between observed and predicted values indicate that our model is too simple; there seems to be interaction between race and the effect of smoking (effect modification).

The xi: prefix also facilitates analyzing models with interactions:

```
. xi: regress bwt i.smoke*i.race
i.smoke          _Ismoke_0-1    (naturally coded; _Ismoke_0 omitted)
i.race           _Irace_1-3     (naturally coded; _Irace_1 omitted)
i.smoke*i.race   _IsmoXrac_#_#  (coded as above)
```

Source	SS	df	MS		
Model	14455540.4	5	2891108.08	Number of obs =	189
Residual	85459758.2	183	466993.214	F(5, 183) =	6.19
				Prob > F =	0.0000
				R-squared =	0.1447
				Adj R-squared =	0.1213
Total	99915298.6	188	531464.354	Root MSE =	683.37

bwt	Coef.	Std. Err.	t	P>|t|	[95% Conf. Interval]	
_Ismoke_1	-601.3654	139.979	-4.30	0.000	-877.5456	-325.1852
_Irace_2	-574.25	199.5008	-2.88	0.004	-967.8674	-180.6326
_Irace_3	-614.5136	138.2182	-4.45	0.000	-887.2198	-341.8075
IsmoXrac~2	250.8654	308.9992	0.81	0.418	-358.7937	860.5245
IsmoXrac~3	544.2957	258.8455	2.10	0.037	33.59039	1055.001
_cons	3428.75	103.0218	33.28	0.000	3225.487	3632.013

The product i.smoke*i.race creates the main-effect dummy variables as before and two product (interaction) variables. The following table shows the values of the dummy and interaction variables for all combinations of the primary variables smoke and race. groups is an unofficial command; see section 10.3 for information on how to obtain it. show(f) displays frequencies; abbrev(13) prevents abbreviation of variable names up to 13 characters:

```
. groups smoke race _I*, sepby(smoke) show(f) abbrev(13) nolabel
```

smoke	race	_Ismoke_1	_Irace_2	_Irace_3	_IsmoXrac_1_2	_IsmoXrac_1_3	Freq.
0	1	0	0	0	0	0	44
0	2	0	1	0	0	0	16
0	3	0	0	1	0	0	55
1	1	1	0	0	0	0	52
1	2	1	1	0	1	0	10
1	3	1	0	1	0	1	12

The significant interaction term _IsmoXrac_1_3 expresses that the effect of smoking on birthweight was significantly different between whites and others; there is effect modification. Now a table of observed and predicted means shows no difference; the regression model fits perfectly; it is "saturated", that is, it includes all possible interaction terms between smoke and race:

```
. quietly xi: regress bwt i.smoke*i.race
. predict pbwt if e(sample)
(option xb assumed; fitted values)
. gen resid = bwt - pbwt
. table smoke, by(race) c(mean bwt mean pbwt mean resid) format(%8.0f)
> stubw(18)
```

race and smoked during pregnancy		mean(bwt)	mean(pbwt)	mean(resid)
1. white				
	0. No	3429	3429	0
	1. Yes	2827	2827	0
2. black				
	0. No	2854	2854	0
	1. Yes	2504	2504	0
3. other				
	0. No	2814	2814	0
	1. Yes	2757	2757	-0

The "perfect" fit does not rule out the importance of other factors not included in the model, and most of the variation in birthweight is not explained by the predictors. The adjusted R^2 (the coefficient of determination) is only 0.12, and the residual plot, figure 13.4, shows a lot of variation around the fitted (or predicted) values. The "strange" pattern is due to the simple fact that there are only six combinations of the predictors:

```
. rvfplot, yline(0)
```

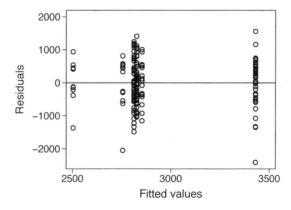

Figure 13.4: Residual-versus-fitted plot

13.2   Logistic regression

In a logistic regression analysis, the outcome is binary and expressed in *odds*, i.e., $p/(1-p)$ (p for probability), and the effect measure is *odds* ratio. Actually, the estimation is performed on a log scale, and at this scale the outcome measure is *logit*, i.e., $\log(p/1-p)$. Logistic regression is the regression model of choice for case–control studies, but it is often used with other designs when the outcome is binary. The logit command displays coefficients on a logit scale, whereas logistic displays odds-ratio estimates; I show only the use of logistic.

The lbw1.dta dataset is from a case–control study: a group of 59 newborns with low birthweight ($< 2,500$ g) were compared with a random sample of 130 normal-weight newborns. This design means that the way the dataset was used in section 13.1 was not quite right; it is unclear what the combined study population represents. Please forgive that abuse of the data. In the dataset, the variable low identifies cases and controls. The distribution and coding of low is shown by tab1:

```
. cd C:\docs\ishr
. use lbw1.dta
(Hosmer & Lemeshow data)
. tab1 low
-> tabulation of low
```

birthweight <2500g	Freq.	Percent	Cum.
0. No	130	68.78	68.78
1. Yes	59	31.22	100.00
Total	189	100.00	

With a dichotomous outcome (birthweight $< 2,500$ g versus $\geq 2,500$ g), the appropriate measure of association in a case–control study is the odds ratio; cc (see section 12.2) calculates the association between maternal smoking and low birthweight:

```
. cc low smoke
```

	Exposed	Unexposed	Proportion Total	Exposed
Cases	30	29	59	0.5085
Controls	44	86	130	0.3385
Total	74	115	189	0.3915

	Point estimate	[95% Conf. Interval]	
Odds ratio	2.021944	1.029092	3.965862 (exact)
Attr. frac. ex.	.5054264	.0282693	.747848 (exact)
Attr. frac. pop	.2569965		

```
                  chi2(1) =     4.92  Pr>chi2 = 0.0265
```

The main result is an odds ratio of 2.02 (95% CI: 1.03, 3.97). A logistic regression gives the same result; however, now the confidence interval is calculated by an approximate method:

```
. logistic low smoke
```

Logistic regression

			Number of obs	=	189
			LR chi2(1)	=	4.87
			Prob > chi2	=	0.0274
Log likelihood = -114.9023 | | | Pseudo R2 | = | 0.0207 |

low	Odds Ratio	Std. Err.	z	P>|z|	[95% Conf. Interval]
smoke	2.021944	.6462912	2.20	0.028	1.080668 3.783083

You should probably ignore two things in the output from `logistic`: the "Pseudo R^2" and the standard errors. Estimation including calculation of confidence intervals is performed on a log scale; to see the "real" SE (ln(OR)), use the `logit` command:

```
. logit low smoke
```
(output omitted)

low	Coef.	Std. Err.	z	P>|z|	[95% Conf. Interval]
smoke	.7040592	.3196386	2.20	0.028	.0775791 1.330539
_cons	-1.087051	.2147299	-5.06	0.000	-1.507914 -.6661886

As with linear regression, you can include continuous and categorical predictors and interactions:

```
. xi: logistic low i.smoke*i.race lwt
```
i.smoke	_Ismoke_0-1	(naturally coded; _Ismoke_0 omitted)
i.race	_Irace_1-3	(naturally coded; _Irace_1 omitted)
i.smoke*i.race	_IsmoXrac_#_#	(coded as above)

Logistic regression

			Number of obs	=	189
			LR chi2(6)	=	22.05
			Prob > chi2	=	0.0012
Log likelihood = -106.31314 | | | Pseudo R2 | = | 0.0939 |

low	Odds Ratio	Std. Err.	z	P>|z|	[95% Conf. Interval]
_Ismoke_1	5.007368	3.030979	2.66	0.008	1.528882 16.40005
_Irace_2	5.100862	3.897479	2.13	0.033	1.140921 22.80508
_Irace_3	4.615637	2.790839	2.53	0.011	1.411087 15.09766
IsmoXrac~2	.6488813	.6833357	-0.41	0.681	.0823695 5.111684
IsmoXrac~3	.2572416	.2307854	-1.51	0.130	.0443284 1.492796
lwt	.9876706	.006333	-1.93	0.053	.9753359 1.000161

When controlling for prepregnancy weight (`lwt`), the association between smoking and low birthweight was OR = 5.007 for white women. For black women, it was 5.007×0.649 = 3.25, and for women of other race it was $5.007 \times 0.257 = 1.29$. For nonsmoking black women versus nonsmoking white women, the odds ratio was 5.10; for smoking women, the corresponding odds ratio was $5.101 \times 0.649 = 3.31$. You can estimate the odds ratio with confidence interval for any combination of predictors by running the `lincom` command after `logistic` (see [R] **lincom**); the commands corresponding to the above calculations are

```
. lincom _Ismoke_1 + _IsmoXrac_1_2

 ( 1)  _Ismoke_1 + _IsmoXrac_1_2 = 0
```

low	Odds Ratio	Std. Err.	z	P>|z|	[95% Conf. Interval]	
(1)	3.249187	2.793182	1.37	0.170	.6026074	17.51923

```
. lincom _Ismoke_1 + _IsmoXrac_1_3

 ( 1)  _Ismoke_1 + _IsmoXrac_1_3 = 0
```

low	Odds Ratio	Std. Err.	z	P>|z|	[95% Conf. Interval]	
(1)	1.288103	.8533323	0.38	0.702	.3516037	4.718977

```
. lincom _Irace_2 + _IsmoXrac_1_2

 ( 1)  _Irace_2 + _IsmoXrac_1_2 = 0
```

low	Odds Ratio	Std. Err.	z	P>|z|	[95% Conf. Interval]	
(1)	3.309854	2.430699	1.63	0.103	.7846956	13.961

Concerning the continuous predictor lwt (mother's prepregnancy weight), the coefficient (0.98767) is the odds ratio for low birthweight per pound of difference in maternal weight. If you want to express this per 50 lb. of difference in maternal weight, the corresponding odds ratio is $0.9876706^{50} = 0.54$; the confidence interval should be treated the same way. lincom gives the same result:

```
. lincom 50*lwt

 ( 1)  50 lwt = 0
```

low	Odds Ratio	Std. Err.	z	P>|z|	[95% Conf. Interval]	
(1)	.5377815	.1724135	-1.93	0.053	.286886	1.008097

You can use predict after logistic to obtain the predicted probability of the outcome for each observation; see [R] **predict**:

```
. xi: logistic low i.smoke i.race
i.smoke           _Ismoke_0-1      (naturally coded; _Ismoke_0 omitted)
i.race            _Irace_1-3       (naturally coded; _Irace_1 omitted)

Logistic regression                         Number of obs   =        189
                                            LR chi2(3)      =      14.70
                                            Prob > chi2     =     0.0021
Log likelihood = -109.98736                 Pseudo R2       =     0.0626
```

low	Odds Ratio	Std. Err.	z	P>|z|	[95% Conf. Interval]	
_Ismoke_1	3.052631	1.12711	3.02	0.003	1.480433	6.294481
_Irace_2	2.956742	1.448758	2.21	0.027	1.131717	7.724832
_Irace_3	3.030001	1.212926	2.77	0.006	1.382618	6.640233

```
. predict plow if e(sample)
(option p assumed; Pr(low))
. table smoke, by(race) c(mean low mean plow) format(%8.4f) stubw(18)
```

race and smoked during pregnancy		mean(low)	mean(plow)
1. white			
	0. No	0.0909	0.1370
	1. Yes	0.3654	0.3264
2. black			
	0. No	0.3125	0.3194
	1. Yes	0.6000	0.5889
3. other			
	0. No	0.3636	0.3248
	1. Yes	0.4167	0.5948

low is the mean of the 0/1-coded variable, i.e., the observed proportion with low birth-weight, and plow is the probability predicted from the regression model for the combination of predictors in each observation; a different model would give different predicted probabilities. Although the observed and predicted probabilities from a case–control study give no meaning beyond the study population, we can compare them.

The model did not give an exact prediction of the risk of low birthweight. For a goodness-of-fit test, we use estat gof after logistic (see [R] **logistic postestimation**). There were six different exposure combinations; the goodness-of-fit test leads us to accept the model:

```
. estat gof
Logistic model for low, goodness-of-fit test
      number of observations =        189
number of covariate patterns =          6
            Pearson chi2(2) =        3.12
              Prob > chi2 =        0.2103
```

If there were many different exposure combinations, a better choice probably would be to use the Hosmer–Lemeshow goodness-of-fit test. We must choose the number of groups:

```
. estat gof, group(10)
```

Unlike regress and logit, logistic does not display a constant (intercept). This omission is sensible for case–control studies where the proportion of cases reflects the study design rather than any true prevalence. In other cases, you may want to see the constant (baseline odds; odds when all predictors are 0). To obtain that, use lincom immediately after logistic:

```
. lincom _cons

 ( 1)   _cons = 0
```

low	Odds Ratio	Std. Err.	z	P>|z|	[95% Conf. Interval]
(1)	.1587319	.0560107	-5.22	0.000	.0794889 .3169727

Despite the header text, 0.1587 is not an odds ratio, but the baseline odds: the odds for the outcome when all predictors are zero—here the odds for low birthweight among white non-smokers. The corresponding probability is $0.1587/(1 + 0.1587) = 13.7\%$. Remember, however, that this was a case–control study, so you cannot generalize absolute risks outside the study population.

13.3   Other regression models

Variations and alternatives to logistic regression

The two commands `logistic` and `logit` (see [R] **logit**) do the same thing; the only difference is that `logit` displays the original coefficients, whereas `logistic` displays the exponentially transformed coefficients, or odds ratios.

If the outcome of interest is not binary, but may take several values, there are a few variations to logistic regression.

If the outcome variable is ordinal, as in (poor/average/good/excellent), see [R] **ologit** (ordered logit estimation).

If the outcome variable is nominal with no natural rank order, as in (Africa/Australia/Asia/Europe, etc.), see [R] **mlogit** (multinomial or polytomous logistic regression).

For matched case–control data, use `clogit` to perform a conditional logistic regression; see section 13.4.

Logistic regression corresponds directly to the case–control design, with odds ratios as the measure of association, but it is often used to analyze cohort data where relative risk is the "natural" measure of association. Binomial regression with the `binreg` command estimates relative risks; see [R] **binreg** and the short example in section 12.1.

Other models

Cox regression and Poisson regression are presented in chapter 14 on survival analysis.

There is a general engine behind most regression models in Stata: generalized linear models; the specific regression commands are modifications to these models. If you are curious, see [R] **glm**. To get an impression of the possibilities, you might take a look at the subject table in the *Quick Reference and Index*. In this chapter, I presented only the analyses most often used in health research.

13.4 Analyzing complex design data

For a nontechnical introduction to analyzing complex design data, I recommend reading chapter 5 in Campbell (2001) or chapters 21 and 30–31 in Kirkwood and Sterne (2003). I will mention two examples: matched case–control studies and repeated observations.

Matched case–control studies: Conditional logistic regression

In matched case–control data we cannot ignore the matching criterion; it must be included in the analysis. In section 12.2, we used the mcc command to analyze 1:1 matched case–control data and saw that the principle is stratification by a variable identifying each matched set. Conditional logistic regression is the corresponding regression model and is performed with the clogit command; see [R] **clogit**. clogit is not restricted to 1:1 matched datasets; there can be any matching ratio, and the ratios may vary between the matched sets.

The lowbirth.dta dataset presented in section 12.2 consisted of 56 pairs of women, matched on age; in each pair, the case woman gave birth to a low-weight child, the control woman to a normal-weight child:

```
. webuse lowbirth.dta, clear
(Applied Logistic Regression, Hosmer & Lemeshow)

. codebook, compact
```

Variable	Obs	Unique	Mean	Min	Max	Label
pairid	112	56	28.5	1	56	Case-control pair id
low	112	2	.5	0	1	Baby has low birthweight
age	112	20	22.5	14	34	Age of mother
lwt	112	57	127.1696	80	241	Mother's last menstrual weight
smoke	112	2	.4107143	0	1	Mother smoked during pregnancy
ptd	112	2	.2232143	0	1	Mother had previous preterm baby
ht	112	2	.0892857	0	1	Mother has hypertension
ui	112	2	.1785714	0	1	Uterine irritability
race1	112	2	.3928571	0	1	mother is white
race2	112	2	.1875	0	1	mother is black
race3	112	2	.4196429	0	1	mother is other

We want to estimate the effect of smoking, race, and age on the risk of low birthweight. Dummy variables for race are already included in the dataset. The matching-set identifier must be specified in the group() option. The or option displays odds ratios rather than the original coefficients:

(Continued on next page)

```
. clogit low smoke race2 race3 age, group(pairid) or
note: age omitted due to no within-group variance.

Iteration 0:   log likelihood = -34.652092
Iteration 1:   log likelihood = -34.598498
Iteration 2:   log likelihood =  -34.59838
Iteration 3:   log likelihood =  -34.59838

Conditional (fixed-effects) logistic regression    Number of obs   =        112
                                                   LR chi2(3)      =       8.44
                                                   Prob > chi2     =     0.0378
Log likelihood =  -34.59838                        Pseudo R2       =     0.1087
```

low	Odds Ratio	Std. Err.	z	P>|z|	[95% Conf. Interval]	
smoke	3.710822	1.849868	2.63	0.009	1.396821	9.858239
race2	1.380827	.8134253	0.55	0.584	.4352195	4.380966
race3	1.888002	.9757447	1.23	0.219	.6856305	5.19894

Interpreting this outcome is straightforward, just like with logistic regression. `clogit`
dropped the matching criterion `age` from the analysis. When you match, you cannot possibly study the effect of the matching criteria.

Repeated and clustered observations

Hosmer and Lemeshow (2000) created a dataset from the low-birthweight data consisting of
487 births among 188 women. A naïve analysis just takes the 487 births as if they were independent observations:

```
. cd C:\docs\ishr
. use clslowbwt.dta
. codebook, compact
```

Variable	Obs	Unique	Mean	Min	Max	Label
id	487	188	93.44969	1	188	Mother id
birth	487	4	1.868583	1	4	Birth number
smoke	487	2	.4004107	0	1	Smoked during pregnancy
race	487	3	1.854209	1	3	Race
age	487	29	26.3963	14	43	Age of mother
lwt	487	131	142.6468	80	272	Prepregnancy weight
bwt	487	447	2840.115	798	5025	Birthweight, grams
low	487	2	.3100616	0	1	Birthweight < 2500g

```
. logistic low age lwt smoke
Logistic regression                          Number of obs   =        487
                                             LR chi2(3)      =      26.40
                                             Prob > chi2     =     0.0000
Log likelihood = -288.32654                  Pseudo R2       =     0.0438
```

low	Odds Ratio	Std. Err.	z	P>|z|	[95% Conf. Interval]	
age	1.048515	.0196192	2.53	0.011	1.010759	1.087682
lwt	.9914686	.0034807	-2.44	0.015	.9846699	.9983143
smoke	2.235806	.4522966	3.98	0.000	1.503968	3.323759

But it is obvious that we do not have independent observations; the birthweights of siblings are correlated, and women have different tendencies to have low-birthweight children. These different tendencies cannot be observed directly but are reflected in the data. Analyzing the data as if we had 487 independent observations leads to an exaggeration of the statistical precision, with standard errors that are too small and confidence intervals that are too narrow.

This is a common situation in health research: women may have more than one child, most people have two legs, and we have up to 32 teeth. The general principle for analyzing these data is to consider the woman, not the births, to be the primary sampling unit; you can do this by using the cluster() option.

```
. logistic low age lwt smoke, cluster(id)
Logistic regression                          Number of obs   =        487
                                             Wald chi2(3)    =      12.26
                                             Prob > chi2     =     0.0065
Log pseudolikelihood = -288.32654            Pseudo R2       =     0.0438

                (standard errors adjusted for clustering on id)
```

low	Odds Ratio	Robust Std. Err.	z	P>|z|	[95% Conf. Interval]	
age	1.048515	.0239779	2.07	0.038	1.002557	1.09658
lwt	.9914686	.0043187	-1.97	0.049	.9830403	.9999693
smoke	2.235806	.6386586	2.82	0.005	1.277286	3.913633

Comparing the two analyses, the point estimates are the same, but the standard errors increased and the confidence intervals became wider. For more information, see [U] **20.14 Obtaining robust variance estimates**.

Stata has a family of commands for analyzing survey data, which are described in the *Survey Data Reference Manual*. One common property of surveys is cluster sampling; here it corresponds to the women's being the primary sampling unit (PSU). Before analysis, the data must be organized by the svyset command:

```
. svyset id
      pweight: <none>
      VCE: linearized
      Strata 1: <one>
      SU 1: id
      FPC 1: <zero>

. svy: logit low age lwt smoke, or
(running logit on estimation sample)

Survey: Logistic regression

Number of strata   =          1          Number of obs    =       487
Number of PSUs     =        188          Population size  =       487
                                         Design df        =       187
                                         F(   3,    185)  =      4.04
                                         Prob > F         =    0.0082
```

low	Odds Ratio	Linearized Std. Err.	t	P>|t|	[95% Conf. Interval]	
age	1.048515	.0239779	2.07	0.040	1.002264	1.0969
lwt	.9914686	.0043187	-1.97	0.051	.9829856	1.000025
smoke	2.235806	.6386586	2.82	0.005	1.272636	3.927931

The result is close to what we found with `logistic` with the `cluster()` option. The `svy:` prefix allows you to analyze complex sampling schemes, such as sampling of school classes, and next sampling of children within each class.

The `xt` family of commands is designed for panel data (repeated observations in a panel of study objects); see the *Longitudinal/Panel Data Reference Manual*. Below, I show a population-averaged model; with options `pa` and `robust`, `xtlogit` gives the following result:

```
. xtlogit low age lwt smoke, i(id) or pa robust

Iteration 1: tolerance = .07354241
Iteration 2: tolerance = .00467504
Iteration 3: tolerance = .00002765
Iteration 4: tolerance = 6.912e-07

GEE population-averaged model         Number of obs      =       487
Group variable:                  id   Number of groups   =       188
Link:                         logit   Obs per group: min =         2
Family:                    binomial                  avg =       2.6
Correlation:            exchangeable                  max =         4
                                      Wald chi2(3)       =     13.49
Scale parameter:                  1   Prob > chi2        =    0.0037

                              (standard errors adjusted for clustering on id)
```

low	Odds Ratio	Semi-robust Std. Err.	z	P>|z|	[95% Conf. Interval]	
age	1.061538	.0210929	3.01	0.003	1.020991	1.103695
lwt	.990815	.0040732	-2.24	0.025	.9828638	.9988305
smoke	2.014735	.5701286	2.48	0.013	1.157032	3.50825

The result differs a bit from what we saw before, but I cannot tell you which is the better choice. The `xt` commands also allow random-effects models, but they are beyond the scope of this book; see Campbell (2001), Dupont (2002), Kirkwood and Sterne (2003), and Hosmer and Lemeshow (2000) for discussions of the merits and weaknesses of different models. The examples in this section used logistic regression, but the principles apply in general: with complex data structures, such as those due to cluster sampling or repeated observations within individuals, the standard models are not valid. It might be a good idea to seek expert advice before you begin designing a study.

14 Incidence, mortality, and survival

14.1 Incidence and mortality

Incidence rates

An incidence rate is estimated by dividing the number of events by the corresponding time at risk. We use the compliance1.dta dataset, which has data on about 555 men aged 64–73 years, who were invited to a screening trial for abdominal aortic aneurysms, and monitored for up to 6 years after randomization; see Lindholt et al. 2005. These data concern a subset of the invited group only; data have been modified to conceal the identity of individuals. We have information on deaths, date of randomization (randate), and date of observation end (enddate). In codebook, the dates are not displayed with a date format but with their numeric value. For information about date variables, see section 5.5.

```
. cd C:\docs\ishr

. use compliance1.dta, clear
(Compliance with invitation to a screening program)

. codebook, compact

Variable   Obs Unique      Mean     Min    Max  Label

id         555    555   6199.575      30  12630  Person number
particip   555      2    .7405405      0      1  Participated
birthdate  555    508  -12484.96  -14235  -9502  Date of birth
randate    555     12    12707.7   12512  14122  Date of randomization
enddate    555    101   14441.18   12597  14609  Date of last observation
died       555      2    .1855856      0      1  Died
```

From the dates, we want to calculate the time at risk in years (risktime), the age at randomization (ranage), this age in 2-year groups (ranagr), and the age at the end of observation (endage). These new variables are included in compliance2.dta. The stset command will be explained in section 14.2.

```
──────────────────────── gen_compliance2.do ────────────────────────
* gen_compliance2.do

cd C:\docs\ishr
use compliance1.dta, clear

generate risktime=(enddate-randate)/365.25
generate ranage=(randate-birthdate)/365.25
generate endage=(enddate-birthdate)/365.25
generate ranagr=2*int(ranage/2)
```

```
label variable risktime "Time at risk"
label variable ranage "Age at randomization"
label variable endage "Age at observation end"
label variable ranagr "Age group at randomization"
label define ranagr 64 "64-65" 66 "66-67" 68 "68-69" 70 "70-71" 72 "72-73"
label values ranagr ranagr

stset risktime, failure(died==1) id(id)

label data "Compliance data -stset- from randomization"
save compliance2.dta, replace
```

We can obtain the number of deaths and the time at risk by typing

```
. use compliance2.dta
(Compliance data -stset- from randomization)

. tabstat died risktime, stat(sum)

    stats │     died   risktime
──────────┼──────────────────────
      sum │      103   2634.032
```

From the 103 deaths and the time at risk of 2,634 years, we can estimate the mortality rate by 103/2,634 years = 0.039 per year, or 39 per 1,000 years. ci estimates the rate and calculates the exact Poisson confidence interval; it is 32 to 47 per 1,000 years:

```
. ci died, exposure(risktime) poisson

                                              — Poisson Exact —
   Variable │   Exposure      Mean    Std. Err.   [95% Conf. Interval]
────────────┼──────────────────────────────────────────────────────────
       died │  2634.032   .0391036    .003853     .0319176    .0474244
```

If we know the number of deaths and time at risk, we can also use the immediate command cii; see section 10.5.

If we have stset the data (see section 14.2), we can obtain an overview of events, time at risk, and incidence rates by stptime. The dd() option lets us decide the number of decimals to display:

```
. use compliance2.dta, clear
(Compliance data -stset- from randomization)

. stptime, by(particip) per(1000) dd(4)
        failure _d:  died == 1
   analysis time _t:  risktime
               id:  id

  particip │  person-time   failures       rate   [95% Conf. Interval]
───────────┼───────────────────────────────────────────────────────────
     0. No │    622.1164         42    67.5115    49.8924     91.3526
     1. Yes │   2011.9151         61    30.3194    23.5904     38.9678
───────────┼───────────────────────────────────────────────────────────
     total │   2634.0315        103    39.1036    32.2363     47.4338
```

We can also display the information for selected time intervals. The argument for the at()
option is a numeric list; see section 4.3.

```
. stptime, by(particip) per(1000) dd(4) at(0(1)5)
           failure _d:  died == 1
     analysis time _t:  risktime
                  id:  id
```

particip		person-time	failures	rate	[95% Conf. Interval]
0. No					
(0	- 1]	137.8782	12	87.0334	49.4271 153.2521
(1	- 2]	124.0424	8	64.4941	32.2533 128.9629
(2	- 3]	116.6441	5	42.8654	17.8418 102.9855
(3	- 4]	109.4901	6	54.7995	24.6193 121.9770
(4	- 5]	97.4237	9	92.3800	48.0667 177.5464
	> 5	36.6379	2	54.5882	13.6524 218.2677
1. Yes					
(0	- 1]	408.8255	5	12.2302	5.0905 29.3833
(1	- 2]	390.9090	13	33.2558	19.3102 57.2728
(2	- 3]	374.6003	7	18.6866	8.9085 39.1971
(3	- 4]	356.4196	15	42.0852	25.3717 69.8086
(4	- 5]	331.5715	15	45.2391	27.2731 75.0401
	> 5	149.5893	6	40.1098	18.0198 89.2796
	total	2634.0315	103	39.1036	32.2363 47.4338

Comparing rates: Stratified analysis

We want to compare the overall mortality rates for those who accepted the screening offer with
those who did not. The question is not whether screening aneurysms affects overall mortality
(aneurysms constitute only a small fraction of all deaths) but whether the general health of the
participants differs from that of the nonparticipants.

However, mortality depends on age, and the tendency to accept a screening offer probably
varies with age, too. To explore the association of participation and mortality with age, we can
use tabstat:

```
. use compliance2.dta, clear
(Compliance data -stset- from randomization)
. tabstat particip died, by(ranagr) format(%6.2f)
Summary statistics: mean
  by categories of: ranagr (Age group at randomization)
```

ranagr	particip	died
64-65	0.80	0.08
66-67	0.83	0.13
68-69	0.70	0.26
70-71	0.67	0.17
72-73	0.69	0.29
Total	0.74	0.19

particip and died are coded 0/1, so the mean (tabstat's default) displays the proportion of subjects who participated and died within the observation period. Participation clearly declines with age. We could test whether the decline is significant, but that is not the point: significantly or not, participation declines with age in our data, and that may confound the comparison of mortality between participants and nonparticipants. To study the participation–mortality association (incidence-rate ratio [IRR]), we use ir (see [ST] **epitab**). To adjust for age at randomization by stratification, we use ir with the by() option:

```
. ir died particip risktime, by(ranagr)
```

Age group at ran	IRR	[95% Conf. Interval]		M-H Weight	
64-65	.3140617	.0744762	1.513131	3.307495	(exact)
66-67	.4926495	.1420931	2.151985	3.341521	(exact)
68-69	.5236575	.228229	1.24793	8.088149	(exact)
70-71	.7504398	.2471127	2.512317	4.137178	(exact)
72-73	.4302365	.2117449	.8811187	12.27482	(exact)
Crude	.4490994	.2982485	.6820111		(exact)
M-H combined	.4913825	.3313807	.7286386		

```
Test of homogeneity (M-H)    chi2(4) =      1.34  Pr>chi2 = 0.8549
```

We can now see the crude mortality-rate ratio estimate (IRR = 0.45), as well as an age-adjusted estimate (IRR = 0.49; 95% CI: 0.33, 0.73). Adjusting for age thus somewhat reduced the contrast between participants and nonparticipants. The test of homogeneity (Pr = 0.85) tells us that there is no evidence of a different association by age (effect modification, interaction).

If we have stset our data (see section 14.2), we can obtain the same analysis by typing

```
. stir particip, by(ranagr)
```

The regression model corresponding to ir is poisson; here we adjust for age at randomization. No wonder that mortality increases with age; the association between participation and mortality is similar to what we found in the age-stratified analysis. Poisson regression is described in more detail in section 14.5.

```
. xi: poisson died particip i.ranagr, exposure(risktime) irr
i.ranagr          _Iranagr_64-72      (naturally coded; _Iranagr_64 omitted)

Iteration 0:   log likelihood = -338.41163
Iteration 1:   log likelihood = -338.40635
Iteration 2:   log likelihood = -338.40635
Poisson regression                          Number of obs   =         555
                                            LR chi2(5)      =       32.23
                                            Prob > chi2     =      0.0000
Log likelihood = -338.40635                 Pseudo R2       =      0.0454
```

died	IRR	Std. Err.	z	P>|z|	[95% Conf. Interval]	
particip	.4889067	.0989234	-3.54	0.000	.3288496	.7268666
_Iranagr_66	1.447485	.599327	0.89	0.372	.6429489	3.258754
_Iranagr_68	2.679351	.9941403	2.66	0.008	1.294797	5.544437
_Iranagr_70	1.663297	.6732149	1.26	0.209	.7523992	3.67698
_Iranagr_72	3.238091	1.161152	3.28	0.001	1.60345	6.539172
risktime	(exposure)					

We can get better results than those from stratifying by age at the start of the observation period; see sections 14.3 and 14.5.

14.2 Survival analysis

In survival analysis, the key variable is the time until an event, such as death, recovery from a fracture, or the duration of the effect of a painkiller. Even if we lose sight of some persons during follow-up (censorings), we can still estimate the proportion of survivors until the end of follow-up, assuming that the risk of those censored does not differ from that of those still under observation. See any good biostatistical or epidemiological textbook, such as Kirkwood and Sterne (2003), for general principles. A more advanced book is Hosmer and Lemeshow (1999). Stata-specific texts are the *Survival Analysis and Epidemiological Tables Reference Manual* and Cleves, Gould, and Gutierrez (2006).

Life table method

The classical method of survival analysis is the life table or actuarial method. `ltable` (see [ST] **ltable**) evaluates the survival function at selected points in time; it also displays the number of persons at risk and the number of events (deaths) and censorings (lost). Although theoretically inferior to the Kaplan–Meier survival estimate (see below), the result comes close if the time intervals are reasonably short. If you can locate only events within prespecified time intervals, you may prefer this method. An example might be persons examined for a disease with annual intervals; you know in which interval the disease occurred but not when.

```
. cd C:\docs\ishr

. use compliance2.dta, clear
(Compliance data -stset- from randomization)

. ltable risktime died, intervals(0(1)5) by(particip)
```

Interval		Beg. Total	Deaths	Lost	Survival	Std. Error	[95% Conf. Int.]	
0. No								
0	1	144	12	0	0.9167	0.0230	0.8579	0.9518
1	2	132	8	5	0.8600	0.0290	0.7915	0.9074
2	3	119	5	1	0.8238	0.0320	0.7503	0.8773
3	4	113	6	3	0.7794	0.0350	0.7012	0.8395
4	5	104	9	3	0.7110	0.0387	0.6273	0.7792
5	.	92	2	90	0.6807	0.0425	0.5893	0.7560
1. Yes								
0	1	411	5	0	0.9878	0.0054	0.9710	0.9949
1	2	406	13	13	0.9557	0.0102	0.9306	0.9719
2	3	380	7	4	0.9380	0.0120	0.9096	0.9577
3	4	369	15	9	0.8994	0.0151	0.8654	0.9252
4	5	345	15	8	0.8598	0.0176	0.8213	0.8906
5	.	322	6	316	0.8284	0.0211	0.7824	0.8655

After 5 years (at the end of interval 4–5), the proportion surviving was 71% among nonparticipants and 86% among participants.

Preparations for survival analysis: The stset command

To prepare for survival analysis (other than with `ltable`), we use the `stset` command; see [ST] **stset**. The `stset` command was included in `gen_compliance2.do`, section 14.1, and resulted in this output:

```
. stset risktime, failure(died==1) id(id)

id:  id
     failure event:  died == 1
obs. time interval:  (risktime[_n-1], risktime]
 exit on or before:  failure

      555  total obs.
        0  exclusions

      555  obs. remaining, representing
      555  subjects
      103  failures in single failure-per-subject data
 2634.032  total analysis time at risk, at risk from t =          0
                              earliest observed entry t =          0
                                 last observed exit t =   5.741273
```

In the `stset` command, we defined `risktime` (time from randomization to end of observation) as the time variable and the code 1 for `died` (failure, in this case death, as opposed to censored at the observation end). We do not really need the `id()` option now, but we will need it later (see `stsplit`, section 14.4). The `stset` output tells us, as we have already seen, that we have 555 observations with 103 failures and a total time at risk of 2,634 years. After we run `stset`, the dataset includes the following variables:

```
. codebook, compact
Variable    Obs Unique       Mean        Min       Max  Label

id          555    555   6199.575         30     12630  Person number
particip    555      2   .7405405          0         1  Participated
birthdate   555    508  -12484.96     -14235     -9502  Date of birth
randate     555     12    12707.7      12512     14122  Date of randomization
enddate     555    101   14441.18      12597     14609  Date of last observation
died        555      2   .1855856          0         1  Died
risktime    555    112   4.746003   .1670089  5.741273  Time at risk
ranage      555    494   68.97373   64.27105  73.79877  Age at randomization
endage      555    508   73.71974   65.51403  78.97057  Age at observation end
ranagr      555      5   67.94595         64        72  Age group at randomization
_st         555      1          1          1         1
_d          555      2   .1855856          0         1
_t          555    112   4.746003   .1670089  5.741273
_t0         555      1          0          0         0
```

`stset` created four new variables, which are used for a number of analyses:

_st   The code 1 means that the observation has valid survival information, such as positive time at risk and a defined status (_d) at observation end.

_d   The code 0 means censoring, and 1 means failure; here it is identical with `died`.

_t   The time at observation end; here it is identical with `risktime`.

_t0   The time at observation start; here it is 0 for everybody.

Once the data are `stset`, several survival analyses can be easily performed.

The Kaplan–Meier survivor function

`sts list` lets us tabulate the Kaplan–Meier survivor function; see [ST] **sts list**. Without the `at()` option, we would get a line for each event. The `failure` option would tabulate 1 − survival instead of survival.

```
. cd C:\docs\ishr

. use compliance2.dta, clear
(Compliance data -stset- from randomization)

. sts list, by(particip) at(0(1)5)
          failure _d:  died == 1
    analysis time _t:  risktime
                  id:  id
```

	Beg.		Survivor	Std.		
Time	Total	Fail	Function	Error	[95% Conf. Int.]	
0. No						
0	0	0	1.0000	.	.	.
1	133	12	0.9167	0.0230	0.8579	0.9518
2	120	8	0.8597	0.0291	0.7910	0.9071
3	114	5	0.8233	0.0321	0.7497	0.8770
4	105	6	0.7784	0.0352	0.6998	0.8387
5	93	9	0.7096	0.0388	0.6256	0.7781
1. Yes						
0	0	0	1.0000	.	.	.
1	407	5	0.9878	0.0054	0.9710	0.9949
2	381	13	0.9556	0.0102	0.9304	0.9718
3	370	7	0.9378	0.0120	0.9093	0.9576
4	346	15	0.8990	0.0152	0.8648	0.9249
5	323	15	0.8593	0.0176	0.8207	0.8902

```
Note:  Survivor function is calculated over full data and evaluated at
       indicated times; it is not calculated from aggregates shown at left.
```

To see the actual number at risk, e.g., after 1 year, use `ltable`. The numbers displayed by `sts list` under the heading `Beg. Total` are slightly different (they are the number at risks at the time of the preceding failure event).

To create a graph with a Kaplan–Meier plot for participants and nonparticipants, the basic command is this simple (the full do-file to create figure 14.1 is available at this book's web site):

```
. sts graph, by(particip)
```

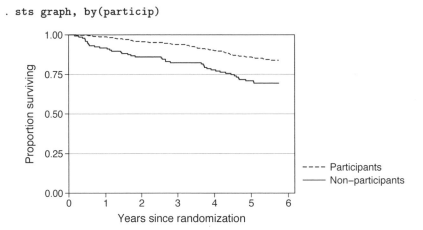

Figure 14.1: Kaplan–Meier plots for two groups

With most subjects surviving, most of the plot area in figure 14.1 is empty. Pocock, Clayton, and Altman (2002) recommend plotting the cumulative incidence proportion (1 − survival) instead; the `failure` option allows that, as shown in figure 14.2. The `ylabel()` option defines the labels at the y-axis; without it, the y-axis would still span from 0 to 1:

```
. sts graph, by(particip) failure ylabel(0(0.05)0.30)
```

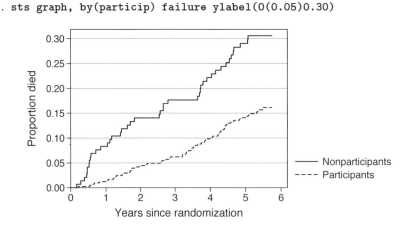

Figure 14.2: Kaplan–Meier plots of cumulative incidence proportion (1 − survival)

Pocock, Clayton, and Altman (2002) also recommend stating the number of persons at risk below the x-axis at selected points in time. There is no easy way to do this, but you can get an imperfect solution, stsatrisk, by typing

```
. findit stsatrisk
```

Log-rank test

The log-rank test compares the observed and expected distribution of events between two or more groups; see [ST] **sts test**:

```
. use compliance2.dta, clear
(Compliance data -stset- from randomization)

. sts test particip
          failure _d:  died == 1
    analysis time _t:  risktime
                  id:  id
```

Log-rank test for equality of survivor functions

particip	Events observed	Events expected
0. No	42	24.23
1. Yes	61	78.77
Total	103	103.00

```
                  chi2(1) =      17.06
                  Pr>chi2 =     0.0000
```

The test can be stratified; here it is stratified by age at randomization:

```
. sts test particip, strata(ranagr)
          failure _d:  died == 1
    analysis time _t:  risktime
                  id:  id
```

Stratified log-rank test for equality of survivor functions

particip	Events observed	Events expected(*)
0. No	42	26.14
1. Yes	61	76.86
Total	103	103.00

(*) sum over calculations within ranagr

```
                  chi2(1) =      13.09
                  Pr>chi2 =     0.0003
```

Several alternative tests are available; see [ST] **sts test**.

14.3   Cox regression

Proportional hazards model

Cox proportional hazards regression estimates hazard ratios; for all practical purposes, they can be interpreted as incidence-rate ratios. Once the data are stset, we can just call stcox with the predictors; see [ST] **stcox**. Here we want to see the association with participation while controlling for age at randomization. The schoenfeld() and basesurv() options are necessary for some of the following analyses (estat phtest and stcurve):

```
. cd C:\docs\ishr

. use compliance2.dta, clear
(Compliance data -stset- from randomization)

. xi: stcox particip i.ranagr, schoenfeld(sch*) basesurv(s)
i.ranagr          _Iranagr_64-72      (naturally coded; _Iranagr_64 omitted)

         failure _d:  died == 1
   analysis time _t:  risktime
                 id:  id

Iteration 0:   log likelihood = -633.74225
Iteration 1:   log likelihood = -618.38181
Iteration 2:   log likelihood =  -617.9045
Iteration 3:   log likelihood = -617.90439
Refining estimates:
Iteration 0:   log likelihood = -617.90439

Cox regression -- Breslow method for ties

No. of subjects =          555                     Number of obs   =        555
No. of failures =          103
Time at risk    =   2634.031508
                                                   LR chi2(5)      =      31.68
Log likelihood  =    -617.90439                    Prob > chi2     =     0.0000
```

_t	Haz. Ratio	Std. Err.	z	P>|z|	[95% Conf. Interval]	
particip	.4844013	.0981015	-3.58	0.000	.325701	.7204295
_Iranagr_66	1.389571	.5758334	0.79	0.427	.6168016	3.130514
_Iranagr_68	2.576273	.9569668	2.55	0.011	1.243969	5.335487
_Iranagr_70	1.58765	.6435182	1.14	0.254	.7173637	3.513744
_Iranagr_72	3.116361	1.120295	3.16	0.002	1.540461	6.304414

The result is similar to that from the corresponding Poisson regression (section 14.1), and the overall interpretation is the same.

The proportional hazards requirement means that the hazard ratio or incidence rate ratio is constant over the time of follow-up. Looking at figure 14.2, we get the impression that during the first year after randomization, the mortality among nonparticipants is much higher than that among participants, while the difference is less marked later (this outcome was actually expected: current ill health may reduce a subject's ability and motivation to participate in a preventive examination). For a graphical assessment of the requirement, use stphplot (see [ST] **stcox diagnostics**):

```
. stphplot, by(particip)
```

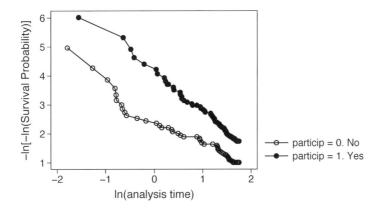

Figure 14.3: Assessment of the proportional hazards requirement with stphplot

When the proportional hazards requirement is fulfilled, the lines are roughly parallel; here we may be in doubt whether the departure is important. This question can be tested formally by running estat phtest (see [ST] **stcox postestimation**) after stcox with the schoenfeld() option; here it was far from significant, so we can accept the proportional hazards assumption:

```
. estat phtest
```
```
       Test of proportional hazards assumption

       Time:   Time
```

	chi2	df	Prob>chi2
global test	3.88	5	0.5667

If we accept the proportional hazards assumption, we can make a graph that corresponds to the assumption, using stcurve after stcox with the basesurv() option:

(Continued on next page)

```
. stcurve, survival at1(particip=0) at2(particip=1)
> ylabel(.7(.05)1, grid)
```

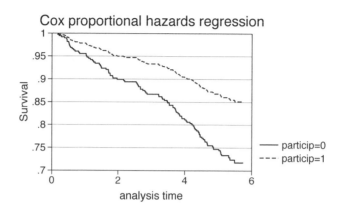

Figure 14.4: Estimated survival curves, based on the proportional hazards assumption

The graph depends on the proportional hazards assumption, but it does not tell us whether the assumption is true.

Using age as the time axis (delayed entry)

Until now, we have analyzed data along a time axis, starting when the subject entered the study (the date of randomization). But the subjects entered the study at different ages, and since age is a strong predictor of mortality, it should be taken into account. We have done that by stratifying or adjusting by the age at randomization, but we can make a more consistent adjustment by using age as the time axis. To do that, we must stset the data again, using the age at observation start (ranage) and end (endage):

```
───────────────── gen_compliance3.do ─────────────────
* gen_compliance3.do

cd C:\docs\ishr
use compliance2.dta, clear

stset endage, enter(time ranage) failure(died==1) id(id)

label data "Compliance data stset with age as time axis"
save compliance3.dta, replace
```

The output from stset follows:

```
. stset endage, enter(time ranage) failure(died==1) id(id)

                 id:  id
      failure event:  died == 1
 obs. time interval:  (endage[_n-1], endage]
 enter on or after:  time ranage
 exit on or before:  failure

─────────────────────────────────────────────────────────────────
      555  total obs.
        0  exclusions
─────────────────────────────────────────────────────────────────
      555  obs. remaining, representing
      555  subjects
      103  failures in single failure-per-subject data
 2634.031  total analysis time at risk, at risk from t =         0
                             earliest observed entry t =  64.27105
                               last observed exit t =  78.97057
```

We defined ranage as the entry time (_t0) and endage as the end of the observation time (_t). The number of events and the time at risk remain unchanged, but the key variables now are

```
. use compliance3.dta, clear
(Compliance data stset with age as time axis)

. codebook ranage endage _*, compact

Variable   Obs Unique     Mean      Min      Max  Label

ranage     555    494  68.97373  64.27105  73.79877  Age at randomization
endage     555    508  73.71974  65.51403  78.97057  Age at observation end
_st        555      1         1         1         1
_d         555      2  .1855856         0         1
_t         555    508  73.71974  65.51403  78.97057
_t0        555    494  68.97373  64.27105  73.79877
```

To tabulate the survivor function with age as the time axis, we use sts list with the at() option. I use 2-year age groups:

```
. sts list, by(particip) at(64(2)80)
            failure _d:  died == 1
        analysis time _t:  endage
     enter on or after:  time ranage
                    id:  id
```

(Continued on next page)

Time	Beg. Total	Fail	Survivor Function	Std. Error	[95% Conf. Int.]	
0. No						
64	0	0	1.0000	.	.	.
66	23	1	0.9444	0.0540	0.6664	0.9920
68	35	0	0.9444	0.0540	0.6664	0.9920
70	52	8	0.7861	0.0682	0.6141	0.8880
72	64	8	0.6856	0.0681	0.5314	0.7982
74	82	8	0.6120	0.0656	0.4709	0.7260
76	45	8	0.5441	0.0626	0.4142	0.6569
78	18	9	0.3985	0.0625	0.2765	0.5175
80	1	0	.	.	.	.
1. Yes						
64	0	0	1.0000	.	.	.
66	99	2	0.9779	0.0155	0.9143	0.9944
68	165	3	0.9560	0.0197	0.8953	0.9819
70	216	7	0.9208	0.0231	0.8610	0.9555
72	194	7	0.8881	0.0254	0.8268	0.9286
74	190	17	0.8129	0.0290	0.7480	0.8627
76	119	13	0.7476	0.0320	0.6785	0.8041
78	46	11	0.6433	0.0414	0.5558	0.7179
80	1	1	.	.	.	.

Note: Survivor function is calculated over full data and evaluated at
       indicated times; it is not calculated from aggregates shown at left.

Now events are put in the age interval when they happened, while each individual's time at risk may be distributed to several age intervals. With age as the time axis, the log-rank test is age adjusted:

```
. sts test particip

        failure _d:  died == 1
  analysis time _t:  endage
  enter on or after:  time ranage
                id:  id
```

Log-rank test for equality of survivor functions

particip	Events observed	Events expected
0. No	42	26.01
1. Yes	61	76.99
Total	103	103.00

	chi2(1) =	13.25
	Pr>chi2 =	0.0003

We can now make an age-adjusted Cox regression. With age as the time axis, we cannot study the effect of age itself, just as a stratified analysis does not let us see the effect of the stratification criterion:

```
. stcox particip

        failure _d:  died == 1
   analysis time _t:  endage
 enter on or after:  time ranage
                id:  id

Iteration 0:   log likelihood = -545.32382
Iteration 1:   log likelihood = -539.49905
Iteration 2:   log likelihood = -539.34835
Iteration 3:   log likelihood = -539.34834
Refining estimates:
Iteration 0:   log likelihood = -539.34834

Cox regression -- Breslow method for ties

No. of subjects =          555              Number of obs   =       555
No. of failures =          103
Time at risk    =  2634.031448
                                            LR chi2(1)      =     11.95
Log likelihood  =    -539.34834            Prob > chi2     =    0.0005
```

_t	Haz. Ratio	Std. Err.	z	P>|z|	[95% Conf. Interval]	
particip	.4875633	.0982525	-3.56	0.000	.3284725	.7237073

Compared with our previous attempts to adjust for age, the results are similar. Letting age be the time axis corresponds to a very fine stratification by age.

14.4   Reorganizing st data

stsplit

We can split an observation into several observations, each describing the experience within a shorter segment of time; see [ST] **stsplit**. We start with the compliance3.dta dataset created in section 14.3; it was stset with age as the time axis:

```
. cd C:\docs\ishr

. use compliance3.dta, clear
(Compliance data stset with age as time axis)

. codebook id _t0 _t risktime _d died, compact
```

Variable	Obs	Unique	Mean	Min	Max	Label
id	555	555	6199.575	30	12630	Person number
_t0	555	494	68.97373	64.27105	73.79877	
_t	555	508	73.71974	65.51403	78.97057	
risktime	555	112	4.746003	.1670089	5.741273	Time at risk
_d	555	2	.1855856	0	1	
died	555	2	.1855856	0	1	Died

For illustration, we can list two selected observations, one that was censored and one that ended in death:

```
. list id _t0 _t risktime _d died if id==249 | id==251
```

	id	_t0	_t	risktime	_d	died
8.	249	73.171799	78.40657	5.234771	0	0. No
9.	251	72.240929	76.035591	3.794661	1	1. Yes

The first person (id 249) had 5.23 years at risk, from age 73.17 until he was censored at age 78.41. The second person (id 251) had 3.79 years at risk, from age 72.24 until he died at age 76.04. With stsplit, we now split each observation in 2-year age groups:

```
──────────────────── gen_compliance4.do ────────────────────
* gen_compliance4.do

cd C:\docs\ishr
use compliance3.dta, clear
stsplit age, at(64(2)80)

* risktime must be re-calculated after splitting.
replace risktime = _t - _t0

label data "Compliance data stsplit 2-year age groups"
save compliance4.dta, replace
```

Now the dataset has been expanded to 1,901 observations, with deaths and time at risk allocated to the proper age intervals:

```
. codebook id _t0 _t risktime _d died age, compact
```

Variable	Obs	Unique	Mean	Min	Max	Label
id	1901	555	6215.619	30	12630	Person number
_t0	1901	501	70.83873	64.27105	78	
_t	1901	515	72.22433	65.51403	78.97057	
risktime	1901	760	1.385603	.0013657	2	Time at risk
_d	1901	2	.054182	0	1	
died	555	2	.1855856	0	1	Died
age	1901	8	70.53866	64	78	

```
. sort id _t0
```

```
. list id _t0 _t risktime _d died if id==249 | id==251, sepby(id)
```

	id	_t0	_t	risktime	_d	died
27.	249	73.171799	74	.8282013	0	.
28.	249	74	76	2	0	.
29.	249	76	78	2	0	.
30.	249	78	78.40657	.4065704	0	0. No
31.	251	72.240929	74	1.759071	0	.
32.	251	74	76	2	0	.
33.	251	76	76.035591	.0355911	1	1. Yes

We can display the number of events and the time at risk for each age interval with `stptime`:

```
. stptime, by(age) per(1000) dd(4)
         failure _d:  died == 1
   analysis time _t:  endage
   enter on or after:  time ranage
                 id:  id
```

age	person-time	failures	rate	[95% Conf.	Interval]
64	129.6399	3	23.1410	7.4635	71.7503
66	307.9316	3	9.7424	3.1421	30.2071
68	465.4429	15	32.2274	19.4288	53.4569
70	507.2169	15	29.5731	17.8286	49.0543
72	529.0705	25	47.2527	31.9291	69.9305
74	437.0404	21	48.0505	31.3293	73.6962
76	220.8980	20	90.5395	58.4122	140.3371
78	36.7912	1	27.1804	3.8287	192.9555
total	2634.0314	103	39.1036	32.2363	47.4338

14.5 Poisson regression

As shown in section 14.1, Poisson is the regression model corresponding to a stratified analysis by `ir`. Think of the dataset as stratified by one or more criteria, each stratum including information on the number of events and the corresponding time at risk.

The `stsplit` dataset `compliance4.dta` generated in section 14.4 is stratified by `particip` (two categories) and `age` (eight categories). We can now perform a Poisson regression adjusted for age. The result is similar to that from the Cox regression in section 14.3: IRR = 0.48 (95% CI: 0.33, 0.72):

```
. cd C:\docs\ishr

. use compliance4.dta, clear
(Compliance data stsplit 2-year age groups)

. xi: poisson _d particip i.age, exposure(risktime) irr

i.age              _Iage_64-78       (naturally coded; _Iage_64 omitted)

Iteration 0:    log likelihood = -464.50154
Iteration 1:    log likelihood = -464.45214
Iteration 2:    log likelihood = -464.45208
Iteration 3:    log likelihood = -464.45208

Poisson regression                            Number of obs    =      1901
                                              LR chi2(8)       =     37.53
                                              Prob > chi2      =    0.0000
Log likelihood = -464.45208                   Pseudo R2        =    0.0388
```

particip	.4834584	.0974273	-3.61	0.000	.3257044	.7176203
_Iage_66	.4220758	.3446237	-1.06	0.291	.0851897	2.091192
_Iage_68	1.376857	.8708156	0.51	0.613	.3985954	4.756036
_Iage_70	1.213949	.7680285	0.31	0.759	.3512947	4.194978
_Iage_72	1.883083	1.151588	1.03	0.301	.5679662	6.243332
_Iage_74	1.885421	1.165099	1.03	0.305	.5615737	6.330088
_Iage_76	3.619279	2.242606	2.08	0.038	1.074469	12.19131
_Iage_78	1.064129	1.22919	0.05	0.957	.1106014	10.23831
risktime	(exposure)					

The first variable in the command (_d) is the event variable; next follow the covariates, while the time at risk is specified in the `exposure()` option.

The same Poisson regression (but not a Cox regression) could also be performed on a collapsed dataset (on `collapse`, see section 9.6). The result is the same; below we list the collapsed dataset with 16 observations after having calculated the mortality rate.

```
. collapse (sum) risktime _d, by(particip age)

. generate mrate = _d/risktime

. list, sepby(particip)
```

	particip	age	risktime	_d	mrate
1.	0. No	64	22.85012	1	.0437634
2.	0. No	66	53.40452	0	0
3.	0. No	68	87.97673	8	.0909331
4.	0. No	70	119.1444	8	.0671454
5.	0. No	72	142.8953	8	.055985
6.	0. No	74	126.2738	8	.0633544
7.	0. No	76	58.84052	9	.1529558
8.	0. No	78	10.73101	0	0
9.	1. Yes	64	106.7898	2	.0187284
	(output omitted)				
16.	1. Yes	78	26.06023	1	.0383727

14.6   Standardization

Standardization methods are examples of stratified analysis, but with weighting methods different from those of Mantel–Haenszel (see section 12.1). In *indirect standardization*, the incidence in the study population is compared with the incidence in a chosen reference population; stratum weights are defined by the distribution of time at risk in the study population, and the result is expressed as SMR (standardized mortality ratio) or SIR (standardized incidence ratio). In *direct standardization*, the reference population is real or hypothetical; it is characterized by its relative age distribution, and standardized rates are calculated using the weights from the reference population.

Indirect standardization

A total of 192 people had a certain operation between 1985 and 1996; they were monitored until they died or until 31 December 2004, whichever came first. The main information is recorded in oppatients1.dta:

```
. cd C:\docs\ishr

. use oppatients1.dta
(Long term mortality after operation)

. codebook, compact

Variable    Obs Unique      Mean       Min       Max  Label

patid       192    192      96.5         1       192  Patient ID
sex         192      2  1.395833         1         2  Sex
bdate       192    192 -8319.198    -19533      4469  Date of birth
begdate     192    190  11561.14      9133     13514  Date of observation start
died        192      2  .2760417         0         1  Died
ddate        53     53   13169.7      9595     16426  Date of death
enddate     192     54  15534.36      9595     16436  Date of death/censoring
begage      192    192  54.42939   16.3258  83.35934  Age at observation start
endage      192    192  65.30749  32.76386  92.18069  Age at death/censoring
```

We want to express the prognosis after operation by comparing the patients' mortality with that of the general Danish population. The dk1991-95.dta dataset holds the age- and sex-specific mortality for Danes during 1991–95, so we decide to use that as the reference.

(Continued on next page)

```
. use dk1991-95.dta, clear
(Data file created by EpiData based on dkk1991-95.rec)

. list, sepby(sex)
```

	sex	agegr	mrate
1.	1. male	0	.00666
2.	1. male	1	.00037
3.	1. male	5	.00021
4.	1. male	10	.00021
5.	1. male	15	.00063
	(output omitted)		
21.	1. male	95	.42985
22.	2. female	0	.0052
	(output omitted)		
38.	2. female	75	.04496
39.	2. female	80	.07604
40.	2. female	85	.1317
41.	2. female	90	.22301
42.	2. female	95	.3662

To proceed, we must stset the data, using age as the time axis (see section 14.2) and next stsplit the observations in age bands corresponding to the file containing the reference rates (see section 14.4). Finally, merge the reference mortality rates to the expanded dataset:

```
─────────────── gen_oppatients2.do ───────────────
* gen_oppatients2.do

clear
cd C:\docs\ishr
use oppatients1.dta

* -stset- data; age is time axis
stset endage, enter(time begage) failure(died==1) id(patid)

* split information in age bands (agegr)
  stsplit agegr, at(0 1 5(5)100)
  label variable agegr "Age band"

* Merge age- and sex-specific reference mortality rates to data
  sort sex agegr
  merge sex agegr using dk1991-95.dta
  drop if _merge<3      // Some age bands in the reference mortality rate file
  drop _merge           // had no match in the actual dataset; they are dropped

label data "Patient data, stsplit and merged with population rates"
save oppatients2.dta, replace
```

The merged dataset, oppatients2.dta, now includes 606 valid observations:

```
. use oppatients2.dta, clear
(Patient data, stsplit and merged with population rates)

. codebook, compact

Variable     Obs Unique      Mean      Min       Max  Label

patid        606    192   89.02805        1       192  Patient ID
sex          606      2   1.389439        1         2  Sex
bdate        606    192  -7784.267   -19533      4469  Date of birth
begdate      606    190   11390.11     9133     13514  Date of observation start
died         192      2   .2760417        0         1  Died
ddate        118     53   13696.07     9595     16426  Date of death
enddate      606     54   15902.48     9595     16436  Date of death/censoring
begage       606    192   52.49657  16.3258  83.35934  Age at observation start
endage       606    207   60.47696       20  92.18069  Age at death/censoring
_st          606      1          1        1         1
_d           606      2   .0874587        0         1
_t           606    207   60.47696       20  92.18069
_t0          606    207   57.03043  16.3258        90
agegr        606     16   56.27063       15        90  Age band
mrate        606     30   .0239183   .00027    .28071  Reference mortality rate
```

strate with the smr() option now calculates SMR; here we see it for each sex:

```
. strate sex, smr(mrate)
        failure _d:  died == 1
   analysis time _t:  endage
  enter on or after:  time begage
                id:  patid

Estimated SMRs and lower/upper bounds of 95% confidence intervals
(606 records included in the analysis)
```

sex	D	E	SMR	Lower	Upper
1. male	34	36.37	0.9349	0.6680	1.3084
2. female	19	9.50	1.9994	1.2753	3.1345

There are other commands that may be useful to estimate SMRs, such as stptime (see [ST] **stptime**) and istdize (see [R] **dstdize**). The istdize command requires considerable data preparation, so strate is much handier.

We can also use poisson to estimate SMR. As preparation, we must calculate the expected number of deaths and use that as the "exposure" instead of the time at risk. With the irr option, poisson does not display the constant, which is the estimate of interest, but we can obtain it with lincom after poisson:

```
. use oppatients2.dta, clear
(Patient data, stsplit and merged with population rates)

. generate pyrs = _t - _t0
(12 missing values generated)

. label variable pyrs "Time at risk"

. replace died = _d
(414 real changes made)
```

```
. gen edied = pyrs*mrate
(12 missing values generated)

. label variable edied "Expected deaths"

. poisson died if sex==2, exposure(edied)
Iteration 0:    log likelihood = -77.492235
Iteration 1:    log likelihood = -77.492235

Poisson regression                          Number of obs   =      236
                                            LR chi2(0)      =     0.00
                                            Prob > chi2     =        .
Log likelihood = -77.492235                 Pseudo R2       =   0.0000
```

died	Coef.	Std. Err.	z	P>|z|	[95% Conf. Interval]	
_cons	.6928325	.2294157	3.02	0.003	.2431859	1.142479
edied	(exposure)					

```
. lincom _cons, irr

 ( 1)   [died]_cons = 0
```

died	IRR	Std. Err.	z	P>|z|	[95% Conf. Interval]	
(1)	1.999371	.4586871	3.02	0.003	1.275306	3.134529

For females, we found the same SMR as with `strate`. With `poisson`, we can also compare the SMRs for males and females; the SMR for females was significantly higher than that for males:

```
. poisson died sex, exposure(edied) irr
Iteration 0:    log likelihood = -225.56715
Iteration 1:    log likelihood = -225.56714

Poisson regression                          Number of obs   =      606
                                            LR chi2(1)      =     6.44
                                            Prob > chi2     =   0.0112
Log likelihood = -225.56714                 Pseudo R2       =   0.0141
```

died	IRR	Std. Err.	z	P>|z|	[95% Conf. Interval]	
sex	2.138617	.6125686	2.65	0.008	1.219893	3.749251
edied	(exposure)					

In the above example, we used Danish mortality 1991–1995 as a reference, although the observations took place during 1985–2004. This example is a bit quick and dirty, and if population mortality changed during the study period, we should use separate reference populations for different calendar periods. The necessary data manipulation corresponds to constructing a Lexis diagram; see Clayton and Hills (1993).

The reference mortality file `dk1981-2004.dta` includes the Danish age- and sex-specific mortality rates for the calendar periods 1981–1985, 1986–1990, 1991–1995, 1996–2000, and 2001–2004:

```
. use dk1981-2004.dta, clear

. summarize
    Variable │      Obs        Mean    Std. Dev.        Min         Max
─────────────┼─────────────────────────────────────────────────────────
        year │      210        1991    7.087964        1981        2001
         sex │      210         1.5    .5011947           1           2
       agegr │      210    45.28571    29.89958           0          95
       mrate │      210    .0496624    .0971473      .00008     .42985
```

To use this information, we should stsplit the patient data first by calendar time and next by age before merging with the reference file. Splitting by calendar time requires that dates be transformed from days since 1 January 1960 to calendar years:

```
————————————————————— gen_oppatients3.do —————————————————————
* gen_oppatients3.do

cd C:\docs\ishr
use oppatients1.dta, clear

* Transform dates to years since year 0.
  gen begyear = 1960 + begdate/365.25
  gen endyear = 1960 + enddate/365.25
  gen byear = 1960 + bdate/365.25

* stset with calendar time as time axis
  stset endyear, enter(time begyear) failure(died==1) id(patid)
* Split observations, one for each calendar time band
  stsplit timeband, at(1981 1986 1991 1996 2001 2006)
* recalculate age at start and end for each timeband
  replace begage = _t0 - byear
  replace endage = _t - byear

* stset with age as time axis
  stset endage, enter(time begage) failure(died==1) id(patid)
* Split observations once more, one for each age band
  stsplit agegr, at(0 1 5(5)100)

* Before merge with the reference file, variable names must match.
  rename timeband year
  sort year sex agegr
  merge year sex agegr using dk1981-2004.dta

* Now calculate expected number of deaths
  gen pyrs = _t - _t0
  gen edied = pyrs*mrate

save oppatients3.dta, replace
```

After we run `merge` by calendar time, sex, and age with the reference mortality file, we can estimate SMR as before using `strate` or `poisson`:

```
. use oppatients3.dta, clear
(Long term mortality after operation)

. strate sex, smr(mrate)

        failure _d:  died == 1
   analysis time _t:  endage
   enter on or after:  time begage
               id:  patid

Estimated SMRs and lower/upper bounds of 95% confidence intervals
(982 records included in the analysis)
```

sex	D	E	SMR	Lower	Upper
1. male	34	33.58	1.0124	0.7234	1.4168
2. female	19	8.83	2.1515	1.3723	3.3730

Direct standardization

In direct standardization, the information in the age strata is weighted by the age distribution in a real or hypothetical population. We might, for example, see a curve of incidence development, adjusted to U.S. 1960 population, or a table of cancer incidence, adjusted to some European or world standard population.

Public-domain data on various standard populations can be downloaded from U.S. National Cancer Institute's site: http://seer.cancer.gov/stdpopulations/. From these data, I created a Stata dataset, `stdpops.dta`, with 11 different standard populations; it can be downloaded from this book's web site.

```
. use stdpops.dta, clear

. tab1 standard

-> tabulation of standard
```

standard	Freq.	Percent	Cum.
1. 2000 U.S.	19	9.09	9.09
2. 1940 U.S.	19	9.09	18.18
3. 1950 U.S.	19	9.09	27.27
4. 1960 U.S.	19	9.09	36.36
5. 1970 U.S.	19	9.09	45.45
6. 1980 U.S.	19	9.09	54.55
7. 1990 U.S.	19	9.09	63.64
8. 1991 Canadian	19	9.09	72.73
9. 1996 Canadian	19	9.09	81.82
10. European	19	9.09	90.91
11. World	19	9.09	100.00
Total	209	100.00	

To see the contents of the European standard, type

```
. list if standard==10, separator(0)
```

		standard	age	pop
172.	10.	European	0. 0	16000
173.	10.	European	1. 1-4	64000
174.	10.	European	5. 5-9	70000
175.	10.	European	10. 10-14	70000
176.	10.	European	15. 15-19	70000
177.	10.	European	20. 20-24	70000
178.	10.	European	25. 25-29	70000
179.	10.	European	30. 30-34	70000
180.	10.	European	35. 35-39	70000
181.	10.	European	40. 40-44	70000
182.	10.	European	45. 45-49	70000
183.	10.	European	50. 50-54	70000
184.	10.	European	55. 55-59	60000
185.	10.	European	60. 60-64	50000
186.	10.	European	65. 65-69	40000
187.	10.	European	70. 70-74	30000
188.	10.	European	75. 75-79	20000
189.	10.	European	80. 80-84	10000
190.	10.	European	85. 85+	10000

`dk1975-2004.dta` is mortality data for Danish males from 7 selected years:

```
. cd C:\docs\ishr
. use dk1975-2004.dta, clear
. summarize
```

Variable	Obs	Mean	Std. Dev.	Min	Max
age	133	40.31579	26.9973	0	85
year	133	1989.857	9.826636	1975	2004
deaths	133	1554.128	1802.25	20	5742
pop	133	135080.1	60133.45	16569	217770

The age distribution changed over the years, so to obtain comparable figures, we perform a direct standardization to the European standard population. First, we create the European standard population file from `stdpops.dta`:

```
_____ gen_std_europe.do _____
* gen_std_europe.do

cd C:\docs\ishr
use stdpops.dta, clear
keep if standard==10
save std_europe.dta, replace
```

The key variables age and pop have the same name in the dataset and the standard population file, and we can use `dstdize`:

```
. cd C:\docs\ishr

. use dk1975-2004.dta, clear

. dstdize deaths pop age, by(year) using(std_europe.dta)
```

```
-> year= 1975
                           ————Unadjusted———  Std.
                             Pop.  Stratum    Pop.
    Stratum      Pop.  Cases Dist. Rate[s]  Dst[P]   s*P
    ————————————————————————————————————————————————————
          0     35625    435 0.014 0.0122   0.016 0.0002
          1    149186    101 0.060 0.0007   0.064 0.0000
          5    202945     95 0.081 0.0005   0.070 0.0000
         10    198652     83 0.079 0.0004   0.070 0.0000
         15    190365    169 0.076 0.0009   0.070 0.0001
         20    193301    234 0.077 0.0012   0.070 0.0001
         25    217770    244 0.087 0.0011   0.070 0.0001
         30    186095    216 0.074 0.0012   0.070 0.0001
         35    151010    281 0.060 0.0019   0.070 0.0001
         40    138301    413 0.055 0.0030   0.070 0.0002
         45    139908    638 0.056 0.0046   0.070 0.0003
         50    148380   1225 0.059 0.0083   0.070 0.0006
         55    133749   1710 0.053 0.0128   0.060 0.0008
         60    130096   2665 0.052 0.0205   0.050 0.0010
         65    109128   3642 0.044 0.0334   0.040 0.0013
         70     80260   4249 0.032 0.0529   0.030 0.0016
         75     53210   4270 0.021 0.0802   0.020 0.0016
         80     29667   3542 0.012 0.1194   0.010 0.0012
         85     16569   3556 0.007 0.2146   0.010 0.0021
    ————————————————————————————————————————————————————
Totals:      2504217  27768       Adjusted Cases:   28806.6
                                     Crude Rate:     0.0111
                                  Adjusted Rate:     0.0115
                        95% Conf. Interval: [0.0114, 0.0116]
```

(*output omitted*)

```
Summary of Study Populations:
     year            N     Crude     Adj_Rate      Confidence Interval
     ————————————————————————————————————————————————————————————————
     1975      2504217  0.011088     0.011503   [  0.011372,    0.011635]
     1980      2529070  0.011938     0.011817   [  0.011687,    0.011947]
     1985      2517078  0.012130     0.011482   [  0.011356,    0.011608]
     1990      2530581  0.012317     0.011196   [  0.011074,    0.011318]
     1995      2573308  0.012151     0.010854   [  0.010737,    0.010971]
     2000      2634126  0.010733     0.009411   [  0.009304,    0.009518]
     2004      2677274  0.010271     0.008656   [  0.008556,    0.008756]
```

The crude rates did not change much over the 30 years, but the adjusted rates did: comparing the crude rates is misleading because of confounding by the changing age structure. However, the standard population is a choice, and with different weights, the results would have been different—although hardly dramatically so.

The standard populations in stdpops.dta are in 5-year age groups, but we might want to use coarser age strata:

```
                          ────────── gen_stdUS1990B.do ──────────
* gen_stdUS1990B.do

cd C:\docs\ishr
use stdpops.dta
keep if standard==7
recode age (0 1=0 "0-4")(5 10=5 "5-14")(15/30=15 "15-34")   ///
    (35/50=35 "35-54") (55/70=55 "55-74")(75/max=75 "75+"),  ///
    generate(age2)
collapse (sum) pop, by(age2)
numlabel, add
rename age2 age

save stdUS1990B.dta, replace
```

```
. list, separator(0)

          age        pop

  1.     0. 0-4      73799
  2.     5. 5-14    141584
  3.    15. 15-34   321459
  4.    35. 35-54   252512
  5.    55. 55-74   157832
  6.    75. 75+      52814
```

The name and coding of the age variable must be the same in your dataset and the standard population file; otherwise, dstdize will not work.

14.7   Some advanced issues

This section discusses some advanced issues that may or may not be important to you. If they are, you can read more in the *Survival Analysis and Epidemiological Tables Reference Manual* or in Cleves, Gould, and Gutierrez (2006). Among topics not described in this book are parametric regression models (see [ST] **streg**) and random-effects models (see [ST] **stcox**).

Time-dependent covariates

In the analysis in section 14.3, we handled age as a time-dependent covariate: as time goes, age changes in a perfectly predictable way, and by letting age be the time axis, we could obtain an age-adjusted hazard ratio.

Also, imagine an event happening at some time during follow-up; the event could affect future risk, but hardly past risk. [ST] **stset** and [ST] **stcox** use the example of heart transplant in patients with serious heart disease. In principle, the solution is to split one observation in two: one censored at the time of a heart transplant and the other starting at the time of the heart transplant and ending with censoring or death. You can do this by using stsplit.

[ST] **stcox** also describes how to handle continuous time-dependent covariates.

Stratified regression

A stratified analysis is relevant when we have designed a matched cohort study, such as one matching by age and sex one or more unexposed persons to each exposed person. Assuming that the persons in a matched set share baseline risk (apart from the exposure), we specify the `strata()` option. Here the variable `setid` identifies the matched sets:

```
. stcox x1 x2, strata(setid)
```

The principle is much the same as in conditional logistic regression, where the `group()` option identifies the matched sets; see section 13.4.

Multiple-failure data

In a standard survival analysis, we look at one event per person, and when the event has happened, it's over; death is the obvious example. Multiple events, such as hospital admissions, are often analyzed with the same model using the time to first admission only, but doing that leaves a lot of useful information unused. On the other hand, multiple admissions cannot be treated as independent events.

The solution described in [ST] **stcox** involves specifying the observations for each person as a cluster by the `cluster()` option. (The `robust` option has the same effect, provided the stset command included the `id()` option.) This example is similar to the repeated-observations problem described in section 13.4:

```
. stcox x1 x2, cluster(id)
```

Competing events

How do we handle deaths from other causes (competing events or risks) if we study mortality from a specific disease? A classical way to handle this is to censor observations at the time of death from any other cause, to estimate the cumulative mortality from this cause if there had been no other causes of death. This situation is counterfactual, but well defined.

The term *cumulative incidence* is used in (at least) two different meanings: the first type is the classical $1 - \text{KM}$ (the Kaplan–Meier survival estimate with deaths from other causes being censored). A second type is an estimate obtained by a modification ensuring that the sum of cause-specific cumulative mortality estimates equals the total cumulative mortality. In the presence of competing risks, the latter cause-specific cumulative incidence becomes lower than the classical estimate; see Farley, Ali, and Slaymaker (2001).

What is "right" depends on the question asked. If you, from the manufacturer's point of view, study the durability (or time to failure) of some kind of prosthesis, death of a patient from unrelated causes obviously prevents you from learning more about this patient's prosthesis, and the classical method of censoring at the time of death answers the question. However, from the patient's perspective, it is relevant to take the risk of dying from something unrelated into consideration; here the question may be whether the prosthesis will fail before the patient dies from something else.

The official Stata st commands are designed to handle competing events the classical way. stcompet estimates the second type of cumulative incidence; see Coviello and Boggess (2004). However, there is no test like a log-rank test available, nor is there any regression model available. stcompet is not an official Stata command; you can find and download it by typing

```
. findit stcompet
```

15 Measurement and diagnosis

15.1 Reproducibility of measurements

Categorical measurements: The kappa statistic

Two radiologists independently classified 85 mammograms (Altman 1991); the results are recorded in rate2.dta. I used numlabel to add codes to the value labels and requested a cross table:

```
. webuse rate2.dta, clear
(Altman p. 403)

. numlabel, add

. tab2 rada radb

-> tabulation of rada by radb
```

Radiologis t A's assessment	Radiologist B's assessment 1. Normal	2. benign	3. suspec	4. cancer	Total
1. Normal	21	12	0	0	33
2. benign	4	17	1	0	22
3. suspect	3	9	15	2	29
4. cancer	0	0	0	1	1
Total	28	38	16	3	85

Among the 85 cases, we find agreement between the two raters in $21 + 17 + 15 + 1 = 54$ cases (63.5%). However, we would expect agreement by pure chance in 30.8% of the cases (we calculate the expected cell values from the marginal distributions). The kappa statistic expresses the amount of agreement beyond the chance expectation; it has the flavor of a correlation coefficient, with 1 indicating perfect agreement and 0 no more than chance agreement. It has been suggested that we interpret kappa values above 0.80 as "almost perfect" and kappa values above 0.60 as "good", but it may be problematic to assign such labels mechanically to a statistic without regard to the problem at hand.

The kap command (see [R] **kappa**) requires that the data structure be wide, i.e., that the two ratings to be compared are in the same observation:

```
. kap rada radb
```

Agreement	Expected Agreement	Kappa	Std. Err.	Z	Prob>Z
63.53%	30.82%	0.4728	0.0694	6.81	0.0000

With an ordinal scale, as in the above example, we see that some disagreements are larger than others, and we may want to let small disagreements (benign versus suspect) have less weight than large disagreements (normal versus cancer). The wgt(w) option automatically weights the agreements according to distance:

```
. kap rada radb, wgt(w)

Ratings weighted by:
   1.0000   0.6667   0.3333   0.0000
   0.6667   1.0000   0.6667   0.3333
   0.3333   0.6667   1.0000   0.6667
   0.0000   0.3333   0.6667   1.0000

              Expected
Agreement    Agreement     Kappa   Std. Err.         Z    Prob>Z

  86.67%       69.11%      0.5684     0.0788       7.22    0.0000
```

You can control distance weights, and it is possible to express the agreement between several raters.

Continuous measurements: Assessing measurement variation

Generally accepted principles for assessing and comparing measurements have been described by Bland and Altman (1986); for a more recent and instructive text, see Bland and Altman (2003). You can find textbook descriptions in Bland (2000) and Kirkwood and Sterne (2003).

The dataset anklebp1.dta contains data on 107 patients with suspected arterial insufficiency in the legs; the dataset includes one leg per patient. Ankle blood pressure was measured twice at the dorsal pedal artery (adp1, adp2) and twice at the posterior tibial artery (atp1, atp2).

```
. cd C:\docs\ishr

. use anklebp1.dta, clear
(Ankle blood pressure data)

. codebook, compact

Variable   Obs Unique      Mean   Min   Max   Label

id         107    107   97.26168    1   194   Patient id
adp1       107     26   116.729    30   195   a.dorsalis pedis (1)
adp2       107     30   117.3364   30   200   a.dorsalis pedis (2)
atp1       107     29   117.9907   30   190   a.tibialis posterior (1)
atp2       107     30   118.3925   30   190   a.tibialis posterior (2)
```

We want to assess the variation of measurement at each site and to compare results from the two sites. Correlation coefficients give us a hint—but not more:

```
. correlate adp1-atp2
(obs=107)
                   adp1      adp2      atp1      atp2

         adp1    1.0000
         adp2    0.9800    1.0000
         atp1    0.9276    0.9298    1.0000
         atp2    0.9291    0.9329    0.9881    1.0000
```

Within each site, the correlation coefficients are high (0.98–0.99); between sites, they are more modest (0.93). A matrix graph gives a nice visual display:

```
. graph matrix adp1-atp2, half ysize(3) xsize(3.1)
```

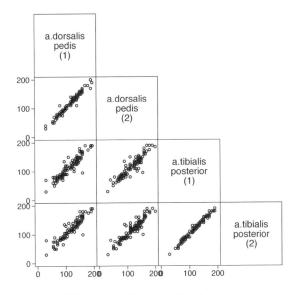

Figure 15.1: Matrix graph comparing four measurements

The matrix graph confirms the impression from the correlation coefficients: there is little variation between same site measurements and somewhat more between different site measurements. Looking at the `codebook` output above, the differences between same site means are small. We now want to express the measurement variation for each site as variances or standard deviations; to do that, we must reshape the data to long format:

(Continued on next page)

```
_____ gen_anklebp2.do _____
* gen_anklebp2.do

cd C:\docs\ishr
use anklebp1.dta, clear
reshape long atp adp, i(id) j(meas)

label data "Ankle blood pressure data; long format"
save anklebp2.dta, replace
```

After we run `reshape` (see section 9.6), the data structure is

```
. list in 1/6, sepby(id)
```

	id	meas	adp	atp
1.	1	1	105	105
2.	1	2	110	105
3.	2	1	110	110
4.	2	2	110	110
5.	4	1	140	150
6.	4	2	130	160

A `oneway` analysis of variance will show us the within-individual variation of measurements on the dorsal pedal artery:

```
. oneway adp id
```

	Analysis of Variance				
Source	SS	df	MS	F	Prob > F
Between groups	271178.271	106	2558.28558	99.09	0.0000
Within groups	2762.5	107	25.817757		
Total	273940.771	213	1286.10691		

```
Bartlett's test for equal variances:  chi2(67) =  33.2114  Prob>chi2 = 1.000

note: Bartlett's test performed on cells with positive variance:
      39 multiple-observation cells not used
```

The within-groups mean square, MS, is the intraindividual variance (25.8), and its square root is the intraindividual variation expressed as standard deviation (5.1 mmHg). We can thus estimate, from the normal distribution, that in about 68% of observations the deviation from the individual mean was within 5.1 mmHg, and in 95% within 10 mmHg. For the `atp` measurements, the intraindividual variation (standard deviation) was 3.9 mmHg.

loneway (see [R] **loneway**) gives some supplementary information:

```
. loneway adp id
                     One-way Analysis of Variance for adp:
                                            Number of obs =       214
                                            R-squared     =    0.9899

        Source           SS        df      MS            F      Prob > F

Between id         271178.27     106    2558.2856      99.09     0.0000
Within id             2762.5     107    25.817757

Total              273940.77     213    1286.1069

            Intraclass        Asy.
            correlation       S.E.        [95% Conf. Interval]

              0.98002       0.00383       0.97250      0.98753

Estimated SD of id effect                            35.58418
Estimated SD within id                                5.081118
Est. reliability of a id mean                         0.98991
         (evaluated at n=2.00)
```

Here we find the estimated variance and standard deviation within id. The intraclass correlation coefficient has the same problems of interpretation as any other correlation coefficient: it depends on the variation both within and between subjects, and when assessing measurement variation we are interested in the within-subjects variation only. The intraclass correlation coefficient and a weighted kappa coefficient can be interpreted much the same way.

15.2 Comparing methods of measurement

The intraindividual variation of the adp and atp measurements was small, so we decide to use the mean of two measurements for comparison of results from the two sites. We generate a modified dataset, anklebp3.dta, including some derived variables:

```
———————————————— gen_anklebp3.do ————————————————
* gen_anklebp3.do

cd C:\docs\ishr
use anklebp1.dta, clear

generate adpmean=(adp1+adp2)/2
generate atpmean=(atp1+atp2)/2
generate ankledif=adpmean-atpmean
generate anklemean=(adpmean+atpmean)/2

save anklebp3.dta, replace
```

We examine the correlation between the mean from each site. A correlation coefficient of 0.94 looks satisfactory, but beware: a correlation coefficient does not tell whether the results from the two sites are identical; if the adp measurements were consistently half the atp measurements, we would get a high correlation coefficient anyway:

```
. correlate adpmean atpmean
(obs=107)

             |  adpmean  atpmean
-------------+------------------
     adpmean |  1.0000
     atpmean |  0.9374   1.0000
```

The most important tool is graphical, and we draw a simple scatterplot with an identity line. We want a square scatterplot, hence the aspectratio(1) option:

```
────────────────────── gph_fig15_2.do ──────────────────────
* gph_fig15_2.do

cd C:\docs\ishr
use anklebp3.dta, clear
set scheme lean1

twoway                                        ///
  (scatter adpmean atpmean)                    ///
  (function y=x, range(0 200) lpattern(l))     ///
  ,                                            ///
  legend(off)                                  ///
  xtitle(atp) ytitle(adp)                      ///
  ysize(2.2) xsize(3) aspectratio(1) scale(1.4)
```

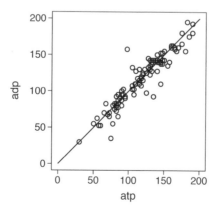

Figure 15.2: Scatterplot with identity line

The line is the identity line (adp = atp), not a regression line. Even in the absence of bias, a regression line would have a slope of less than one due to regression toward the mean. We can compare means with a paired t test and become satisfied:

```
. ttest adpmean==atpmean

Paired t test
```

Variable	Obs	Mean	Std. Err.	Std. Dev.	[95% Conf. Interval]	
adpmean	107	117.0327	3.457543	35.76511	110.1778	123.8876
atpmean	107	118.1916	3.400341	35.1734	111.4501	124.9331
diff	107	-1.158879	1.215053	12.5686	-3.567839	1.250082

```
        mean(diff) = mean(adpmean - atpmean)                    t =  -0.9538
    Ho: mean(diff) = 0                         degrees of freedom =      106

    Ha: mean(diff) < 0          Ha: mean(diff) != 0          Ha: mean(diff) > 0
    Pr(T < t) = 0.1712      Pr(|T| > |t|) = 0.3424          Pr(T > t) = 0.8288
```

In a Bland–Altman plot, the difference between two measurements is plotted against their mean. The procedure does not exist in official Stata, but let's see if there are any user-written commands by typing

```
. findit bland altman
```

This command leads to the following information:

```
STB-55   sbe33 . . . . Comparing several methods of measuring the same quantity
         (help baplot, bagroup, bamat, sdpair if installed) . . . . . P. Seed
         5/00    pp.2--9; STB Reprints Vol 10, pp.73--82
         commands implementing the Bland-Altman approach to comparing
         two or more measurement methods;  also alternative command to
         sdtest based on Pitman's method giving confidence intervals
         for variance ratios of paired data
```

After clicking on sbe33, installing the package, and reading the help file, we can examine the result:

```
. use anklebp3.dta, clear
(Ankle blood pressure data)

. baplot adpmean atpmean

Bland-Altman comparison of adpmean and atpmean
Limits of agreement (Reference Range for difference): -26.296 to 23.978
Mean difference: -1.159 (CI -3.568 to  1.250)
Range : 30.000 to 191.250
Pitman's Test of difference in variance: r =  0.048, n = 107, p = 0.625
```

The mean difference gives the same result as the paired t test above; it was not significant: -1.16 mmHg (95% CI: -3.57, 1.25). The *limits of agreement* describe a 95% reference range or prediction interval (-26.3, 24.0) for the difference between the two measurements; if we assume a normal distribution, we expect 95% of the observed differences to lie within this interval. We also get a graph in the old Stata style (not shown), but with the output information, it is not too difficult to create one using modern graphics:

```
────────────── gph_fig15_3.do ──────────────
* gph_fig15_3.do

cd C:\docs\ishr
use anklebp3.dta, clear

twoway                                    ///
  (scatter ankledif anklemean)            ///
  ,                                       ///
  ytitle("Difference")                    ///
  xtitle("Average")                       ///
  ylabel(-50(25)50)                       ///
  yline(-1.159, lpattern(l))              ///
  yline(-26.296 23.978, lpattern(dash))   ///
  ysize(2.2) xsize(3.1) scale(1.4)
```

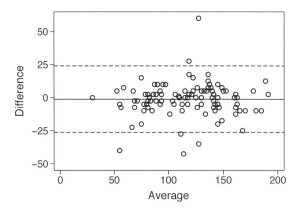

Figure 15.3: Bland–Altman plot of difference versus average of two measurements

The Bland–Altman plot can be used to examine whether the measurement differences depend on the blood pressure level (similarly to examining a residual plot to assess heteroskedasticity; section 13.1). This seems not to be the case. The mean difference is close to 0, so there is no systematic difference in results from the two sites. In 95% of paired observations, the difference was within 25 mmHg, and the remaining question is whether this finding is satisfactory from a clinical point of view.

The analysis performed does not permit us to determine which artery gives the most valid results, but comparing the intraindividual variations might give a clue. sdpair (downloaded with the package for Bland–Altman analysis) lets us compare the standard deviations between differences (dadp and datp):

```
. use anklebp1.dta, clear
(Ankle blood pressure data)

. gen dadp = adp1-adp2

. gen datp = atp1-atp2

. sdpair datp dadp
Pitman's variance ratio test between datp and dadp:

Ratio of Standard deviations = 0.7592
95% Confidence Interval 0.6265 to 0.9200
t = -2.862, df = 105, p =  0.005
```

Pitman's variance-ratio test shows that the intraindividual variation is significantly smaller for atp than for adp, and we can interpret this as atp being the most precise measurement. Whether the differences are clinically important is another question, and we would like to compare with a clinically meaningful external criterion, a "gold standard". This question will be addressed in more detail in section 15.3.

15.3 Using tests for diagnosis

If we have a "gold standard", i.e., a chosen criterion of truth, we can estimate the agreement between a test and the truth it is meant to measure. My recommended reading is Sackett et al. (1991). A statistically more advanced text is given by Pepe (2003).

The data used in this section are partly constructed, and they should not be used as evidence when considering diagnosis of renal artery stenosis. The ras.dta dataset is a modified version of the data used by Habbema et al. (2002): 437 patients suspected of renal-artery stenosis had angiography performed, and the result of the angiography was considered the criterion of truth. However, angiography is an invasive procedure, carrying some risk to the patient, and the question was whether less-risky and less-expensive procedures could be used for diagnostic purposes and reduce the number of patients exposed to angiography. The dataset includes the following variables:

```
. cd C:\docs\ishr

. use ras.dta, clear
(Diagnosis of renal artery stenosis)

. codebook, compact
```

Variable	Obs	Unique	Mean	Min	Max	Label
patid	437	437	219	1	437	Patient ID
stenosis	437	2	.228833	0	1	Stenosis at angiography
renogram	437	2	.2379863	0	1	Abnormal renography
crea	437	102	93.12815	51	189	S-creatinine, micro-mol/L
creagrp	437	10	88.09382	51	151	S-creatinine, grouped

Dichotomous tests

The renogram is a noninvasive imaging test; it can be positive, indicating possible renal ischemia, or negative (things are no doubt more complicated than that). First, let's look at a cross table between angiography and renography results:

```
. tab2 renogram stenosis, col

-> tabulation of renogram by stenosis
```

```
┌─────────────────────────────┐
│ Key                         │
├─────────────────────────────┤
│            frequency        │
│    column percentage        │
└─────────────────────────────┘
```

Abnormal renography	Stenosis at angiography 0. no	1. yes	Total
0. no	304 90.21	29 29.00	333 76.20
1. yes	33 9.79	71 71.00	104 23.80
Total	337 100.00	100 100.00	437 100.00

Among the 437 patients, 100 (23%) had stenosis at angiography. Among those with stenosis 71% had an abnormal renography; among other patients, it was 10%.

To estimate the sensitivity and specificity of renography in diagnosing renal-artery stenosis, we can use `ci` with the `binomial` option (see section 10.5 and [R] **ci**):

```
. by stenosis, sort: ci renogram, binomial
```

```
-> stenosis = 0. no
```

Variable	Obs	Mean	Std. Err.	— Binomial Exact — [95% Conf. Interval]	
renogram	337	.0979228	.0161901	.068368	.134768

```
-> stenosis = 1. yes
```

Variable	Obs	Mean	Std. Err.	— Binomial Exact — [95% Conf. Interval]	
renogram	100	.71	.0453762	.610734	.7964258

The sensitivity is estimated to be 0.71 (95% CI: 0.61, 0.80), and the specificity to be 1 − 0.098 = 0.90 (95% CI: 0.87, 0.93). In the same manner, we could estimate the positive and negative predictive values in this patient population by using the command

```
. by renogram, sort: ci stenosis, binomial
```

Official Stata has no commands with the specific purpose to estimate sensitivity, specificity and predictive values, but with

```
. findit sensitivity specificity
```

we locate

```
SJ-4-4  sbe36_2 . . . . . . . . . . . . . . . . . Software update for diagt
        (help diagt if installed) . . . . . . . . . P. T. Seed and A. Tobias
        Q4/04   SJ 4(4):490
        new options added to diagt
```

Information on this procedure was published in the *Stata Journal*, Volume 4, Number 4. Click the link sbe36_2 to install diagt and then read the help file. To estimate the parameters of interest, type

```
. diagt stenosis renogram
```

Stenosis at angiograph y	Abnormal renography		Total
	Pos.	Neg.	
Abnormal	71	29	100
Normal	33	304	337
Total	104	333	437

True abnormal diagnosis defined as stenosis = 1 (labelled 1. yes)

			[95% Confidence Interval]	
Prevalence	Pr(A)	23%	19%	27.1%
Sensitivity	Pr(+|A)	71%	61.1%	79.6%
Specificity	Pr(-|N)	90.2%	86.5%	93.2%
ROC area	(Sens. + Spec.)/2	.806	.759	.853
Likelihood ratio (+)	Pr(+|A)/Pr(+|N)	7.25	5.12	10.3
Likelihood ratio (-)	Pr(-|A)/Pr(-|N)	.321	.236	.438
Odds ratio	LR(+)/LR(-)	22.6	12.9	39.5
Positive predictive value	Pr(A|+)	68.3%	58.4%	77.1%
Negative predictive value	Pr(N|-)	91.3%	87.7%	94.1%

The table reports sensitivity and specificity and the ROC area. The (rather unusual) ROC curve can be shown by

```
. roctab stenosis renogram, graph
```

An ROC area of 1 means perfect agreement, and 0.5 means that there is no more than random agreement. Sensitivity and specificity are combined in likelihood ratios for positive and negative test results, and the ratio between these is the odds ratio from the 2×2 table.

The positive and negative predictive value estimates are valid for the actual study population and for similar patient populations with the same prior probability of disease (disease prevalence 23%). We may now ask: how would the test perform in a population with a different prior risk of disease, such as 10%? This can be examined by including the prev() option in the diagt command:

```
. diagt stenosis renogram, prev(10%)
```

(output omitted)

			[95% Confidence Interval]	
Prevalence	Pr(A)	10%	——— (given) ———	
Sensitivity	Pr(+|A)	71%	61.1%	79.6%
Specificity	Pr(-|N)	90.2%	86.5%	93.2%
ROC area	(Sens. + Spec.)/2	.806	.759	.853
Likelihood ratio (+)	Pr(+|A)/Pr(+|N)	7.25	5.12	10.3
Likelihood ratio (-)	Pr(-|A)/Pr(-|N)	.321	.236	.438
Odds ratio	LR(+)/LR(-)	22.6	12.9	39.5
Positive predictive value	Pr(A|+)	44.6%	36.3%	53.3% (lr)
Negative predictive value	Pr(N|-)	96.6%	95.4%	97.4% (lr)
Pre-test odds	prev/(1-prev)	.111	——— (given) ———	
Post-test odds (+)	Pr(A|+)/(1-Pr(A|+))	.806	.569	1.14 (lr)
Post-test odds (-)	Pr(A|-)/(1-Pr(A|-))	.0357	.0486	.0262 (lr)

(lr) Values and confidence intervals are based on likelihood
      ratios, assuming that the prevalence is known exactly.

As expected, the positive predictive value decreased and the negative predictive value increased when applying the test in a population with lower prior risk of disease. The calculations depend on sensitivity and specificity being the same in different patient populations, and that assumption may be questioned; see e.g., Sackett and Haynes (2002).

Continuous tests

With continuous tests, e.g., biochemical concentrations, sensitivity and specificity can be estimated for a chosen cutpoint; typically there is a trade-off so that moving the cutpoint to increase sensitivity reduces specificity and vice versa. ROC (receiver operating characteristic) analysis can give an overall estimate of the discriminatory power of a continuous test. See [R] **roc** for a description of the family of commands useful for ROC analysis.

The main parameter of interest is the area under the curve. For a perfect test, the area is 1; for a test with no association between test result and disease status, the area is 0.5. Using crea (serum creatinine) as the test, roctab calculates the area under the curve; it is 0.70 (95% CI: 0.64, 0.76):

```
. use ras.dta
(Diagnosis of renal artery stenosis)

. roctab stenosis crea, summary graph
```

	ROC		—Asymptotic Normal—	
Obs	Area	Std. Err.	[95% Conf. Interval]	
437	0.7009	0.0309	0.64034	0.76153

roctab with the graph option displays the ROC curve; see the full command at this book's web site (gph_fig15_4.do).

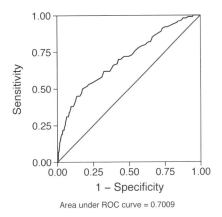

Area under ROC curve = 0.7009

Figure 15.4: ROC curve: Serum creatinine as predictor of renal artery stenosis

The ROC curve does not display test values, but the `detail` option creates a table. To avoid a huge table, we used the grouped variable `creagrp`. We cannot, however, determine the optimal cutpoint without considering health and cost consequences of false negative and false positive test results.

```
. roctab stenosis creagrp, detail
Detailed report of Sensitivity and Specificity
```

Cut point	Sensitivity	Specificity	Correctly Classified	LR+	LR-
(>= 51. -60)	100.00%	0.00%	22.88%	1.0000	
(>= 61. 61-70)	99.00%	5.64%	27.00%	1.0492	0.1774
(>= 71. 71-80)	95.00%	16.32%	34.32%	1.1353	0.3064
(>= 81. 81-90)	82.00%	36.20%	46.68%	1.2853	0.4972
(>= 91. 91-100)	70.00%	57.27%	60.18%	1.6382	0.5238
(>= 101. 101-110)	53.00%	78.34%	72.54%	2.4467	0.6000
(>= 111. 111-120)	38.00%	90.50%	78.49%	4.0019	0.6850
(>= 121. 121-130)	31.00%	93.47%	79.18%	4.7486	0.7382
(>= 131. 131-150)	22.00%	96.14%	79.18%	5.7031	0.8113
(>= 151. 151+)	11.00%	98.52%	78.49%	7.4140	0.9034
(> 151. 151+)	0.00%	100.00%	77.12%		1.0000

Obs	ROC Area	Std. Err.	—Asymptotic Normal—[95% Conf. Interval]	
437	0.7028	0.0309	0.64219	0.76333

The `roccomp` command lets us compare two or more tests or compare subgroups of observations. Here we compare the creatinine-stenosis association among patients with and without abnormal renogram:

```
. roccomp stenosis crea, by(renogram) summary graph
                            ROC                    —Asymptotic Normal—
    renogram       Obs      Area     Std. Err.    [95% Conf. Interval]

    0              333     0.5698      0.0473      0.47709      0.66254
    1              104     0.6921      0.0588      0.57683      0.80730

Ho: area(0) = area(1)
      chi2(1) =    2.62         Prob>chi2 =    0.1053
```

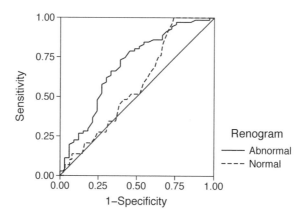

Figure 15.5: ROC curves for creatinine among patients with abnormal and normal renogram

You can find the full graph command (`gph_fig15_5.do`) at this book's web site.

It seems from the table and the graph that there was almost no association between creatinine level and stenosis among patients with a normal renogram, while there was a significant association among patients with an abnormal renogram. However, the areas under the curve were not significantly different ($Pr = 0.11$). In both groups the area under the curve was smaller than in the overall analysis (figure 15.4). Serum creatinine and renography results are not independent, and with knowledge of the renography result, the discriminatory power of serum creatinine diminishes.

15.4 Combining test results

In section 15.3, we saw that both the renogram result and the serum creatinine level contributed to the prediction of stenosis. The likelihood ratio for an abnormal renogram was 7.25, and the likelihood ratio for serum creatinine ≥ 111 μmol/L was 4.00, and we might want to combine the information. The prior odds of stenosis were $100/337 = 0.297$, and the odds of stenosis in a patient with an abnormal renogram and serum creatinine ≥ 111 μmol/L are $0.297 \times 7.25 \times 4.00 = 8.613$; the corresponding probability is $8.613/9.613 = 0.90$.

This calculation ignores the fact that renography result and serum creatinine are not independent. To allow for dependence, perform a logistic regression:

```
. cd C:\docs\ishr

. use ras.dta
(Diagnosis of renal artery stenosis)

. logistic stenosis renogram crea
Logistic regression                             Number of obs   =        437
                                                LR chi2(2)      =     152.91
                                                Prob > chi2     =     0.0000
Log likelihood = -158.59076                     Pseudo R2       =     0.3253
```

stenosis	Odds Ratio	Std. Err.	z	P>|z|	[95% Conf. Interval]	
renogram	17.68998	5.228973	9.72	0.000	9.911079	31.57429
crea	1.017621	.005813	3.06	0.002	1.006291	1.029078

The `lroc` command after `logistic` draws a ROC curve and calculates the area under the curve:

```
. lroc
Logistic model for stenosis

number of observations =        437
area under ROC curve   =     0.8377
```

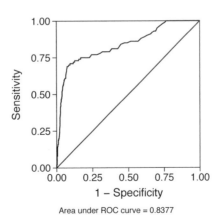

Area under ROC curve = 0.8377

Figure 15.6: ROC curve utilizing the combined results from renography and serum creatinine

When we compare it with the areas found in section 15.3 for renography (0.806) and serum creatinine (0.701), the combination of tests has greater discriminatory power. However, `lroc` does not display the confidence interval for the area; to obtain that, we use `predict` after `logistic` and use the predicted probability (prob) as input to `roctab`. About `predict`, see section 13.1.

```
. predict prob if e(sample)
(option p assumed; Pr(stenosis))
. roctab stenosis prob, summary
```

| | ROC | | —Asymptotic Normal— | |
Obs	Area	Std. Err.	[95% Conf. Interval]	
437	0.8377	0.0252	0.78818	0.88713

An ROC curve does not show the actual test values, but we may use `adjust` after `logistic` (see section 13.2) to get the probability of disease with a given combination of test values. For patients with a serum creatinine of 70 μmol/L, the probability of stenosis with normal and abnormal renograms is estimated by typing

```
. quietly logistic stenosis renogram crea
. adjust crea=70, by(renogram) pr ci
```

```
       Dependent variable: stenosis     Command: logistic
    Covariate set to value: crea = 70
```

Abnormal renograph y	pr	lb	ub
0. no	.061929	[.039741	.095274]
1. yes	.538711	[.401669	.670141]

```
       Key: pr      = Probability
            [lb , ub] = [95% Confidence Interval]
```

With one continuous and one categorical test, we can graph the predicted probability (prob) obtained by `predict` for any combination of test results. The data must be sorted by `crea` before graphing:

```
. sort crea
. twoway (line prob crea if renogram==1)(line prob crea if renogram==0)
```

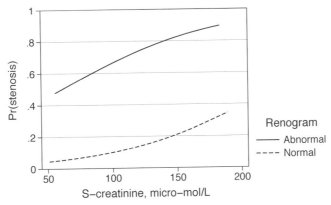

Figure 15.7: Predicted probability of stenosis, by renography and serum creatinine results

If we—considering the benefits, risks and costs associated with angiography—decide that angiography is indicated if the predicted probability of stenosis is at least 10%, the rule should be that angiography be offered to all patients with an abnormal renogram and to patients with serum creatinine > 100 μmol/L. This would lead to angiography being offered to 181 (41%) of the initially suspected patients, with a positive predictive value of 43% and a negative predictive value of 91%:

```
. generate p10 = prob>0.10 if prob<.

. diagt stenosis p10
```

Stenosis at angiography	p10 Pos.	Neg.	Total
Abnormal	78	22	100
Normal	103	234	337
Total	181	256	437

True abnormal diagnosis defined as stenosis = 1 (labelled 1. yes)

			[95% Confidence Interval]	
Prevalence	Pr(A)	23%	19%	27.1%
Sensitivity	Pr(+|A)	78%	68.6%	85.7%
Specificity	Pr(-|N)	69.4%	64.2%	74.3%
ROC area	(Sens. + Spec.)/2	.737	.69	.785
Likelihood ratio (+)	Pr(+|A)/Pr(+|N)	2.55	2.11	3.09
Likelihood ratio (-)	Pr(-|A)/Pr(-|N)	.317	.218	.461
Odds ratio	LR(+)/LR(-)	8.05	4.77	13.6
Positive predictive value	Pr(A|+)	43.1%	35.8%	50.6%
Negative predictive value	Pr(N|-)	91.4%	87.3%	94.5%

16 Miscellaneous

16.1 Random samples, simulations

Random-number functions

The fundamental random-number function in Stata is `uniform()` (no arguments, just empty parentheses); it creates "pseudorandom" numbers uniformly distributed in the interval 0–1:

```
. generate y=uniform()
```

The term "pseudorandom" refers to the fact that no computer program can generate number sequences that are truly random, but you can generate number sequences that exhibit no predictable pattern.

The `uniform()` function can be combined with other functions and operators (see [D] **functions**) to obtain random numbers with a desired distribution:

`. generate y = invnormal(uniform())`	Normal distribution, mean $= 0$, SD $= 1$
`. generate y = 10 + 2*invnormal(uniform())`	Normal distribution, mean $= 10$, SD $= 2$

If you run the same command twice it will yield *different* number sequences. If you need to reproduce the same series of "random" numbers, initialize the seed (a large integer used for the initial calculations):

```
. set seed 654321
```

Random samples and randomization

You can use `sample` to select a random sample of your dataset; see [D] **sample**:

`. sample 10`	Selects an approximately 10% random sample.
`. sample 53, count`	Selects exactly 53 observations at random.

You may assign observations randomly to two treatments by typing

```
. generate y=uniform()
. generate treat=1
. replace treat=0 if y<0.5
```

The same result could be obtained with one command. `uniform()>0.5` evaluates to 1 if it is true; otherwise it evaluates to 0:

```
. generate treat = uniform()>0.5
```

You can sort your observations in random sequence:

```
. generate y=uniform()
. sort y
```

Generating artificial datasets

You can use `set obs` to create empty observations. The following sequence creates a file with 10,000 observations used to study the behavior of the difference (`dif`) between two measurements (`x1`, `x2`), given information about components of variance (`sdwithin`, `sdbetw`):

```
. clear
. set obs 10000
obs was 0, now 10000
. generate sdbetw = 20
. generate sdwithin = 10
. generate x0 = 50 + sdbetw * invnormal(uniform())
. generate x1 = x0 + sdwithin * invnormal(uniform())
. generate x2 = x0 + sdwithin * invnormal(uniform())
. generate dif = x2 - x1
. summarize
```

Variable	Obs	Mean	Std. Dev.	Min	Max
sdbetw	10000	20	0	20	20
sdwithin	10000	10	0	10	10
x0	10000	49.98802	20.01317	-28.37861	122.8318
x1	10000	49.97299	22.3201	-35.09606	134.0619
x2	10000	49.91645	22.32367	-36.9789	136.4258
dif	10000	-.0565401	14.23174	-62.03582	51.71009

However, since `sdbetw` and `sdwithin` are constants, you do not need to create them as variables; it is more efficient to define them as local macros (see section 17.2), and part of the above commands could be

```
. ...
. local SDB = 20
. local SDW = 10
. generate x0 = 50 + 'SDB' * invnormal(uniform())
. generate x1 = x0 + 'SDW' * invnormal(uniform())
. generate x2 = x0 + 'SDW' * invnormal(uniform())
. ...
```

See another example of artificial data in section 11.8 (the `twoway rspike` graph).

Advanced simulations

With `simulate` we can set up complex Monte Carlo simulations; see [R] **simulate**. You might also want to study [R] **bootstrap**, [R] **jackknife**, and [R] **permute** for more advanced topics.

16.2 Sample size and study power

Sample-size and study-power estimation are prestudy activities: what are the consequences of different decisions and assumptions for sample size and study power? The immediate command `sampsi` lets us calculate the required sample size or the power of a study; see [R] **sampsi**.

We must make the following decisions:

- The desired significance level (α); the default is 0.05.
- The minimum relevant contrast that you do not want to miss, expressed as study group means or proportions.
- For sample size estimation: the desired power ($1 - \beta$). The default is 0.90.
- For power estimation: sample sizes.

With comparison of means, you must also make an *assumption*: the assumed standard deviation in each sample.

Below are short examples for the four main scenarios:

Comparison of	Sample size estimation	Power estimation
Proportions	`sampsi 0.4 0.5`	`sampsi 0.4 0.5, n(60)`
Means	`sampsi 50 60, sd(8)`	`sampsi 50 60, sd(8) n(60)`

Further options are available:

Situation	Options	Sample size estimation Proportions	Sample size estimation Means	Power estimation Proportions	Power estimation Means
Significance level; default: 0.05	`alpha(0.01)`	+	+	+	+
Power; default: 0.90	`power(0.95)`	+	+		
Unequal sample sizes; ratio = n2/n1	`ratio(2)`	+	+		
Unequal sample sizes	`n1(40) n2(80)`			+	+
Unequal SDs	`sd1(6) sd2(9)`		+		+

Example: Sample-size estimation for comparison of means, unequal SDs, and sample sizes:

```
. sampsi 50 60, sd1(14) sd2(10) ratio(2)
Estimated sample size for two-sample comparison of means
Test Ho: m1 = m2, where m1 is the mean in population 1
                    and m2 is the mean in population 2
Assumptions:
           alpha =    0.0500   (two-sided)
           power =    0.9000
              m1 =        50
              m2 =        60
             sd1 =        14
             sd2 =        10
           n2/n1 =      2.00
Estimated required sample sizes:
              n1 =        26
              n2 =        52
```

sampsi also handles trials with repeated measurements; see [R] **sampsi**. Creative users have created programs for sample-size and power calculations for special cases; type

```
. findit sample size
```

One of the hits is a paper by Newson (2004) with a description of the versatile powercal command.

16.3   Other analyses

Meta-analysis

Stata has not produced commands specifically aimed at meta-analysis. However, a British group has written several commands aimed at meta-analysis; see Egger, Davey-Smith, and Altman (2001). A revised version of the book's chapter on meta-analysis with Stata can (at least it could as of January 2006) be downloaded from http://www.systematicreviews.com.

Classifying diseases

Facilities for handling diagnostic and procedure codes from ICD-9 (International Classification of Diseases, Ninth Revision) are available with the icd9 and icd9p commands; see [D] **icd9**. Similar facilities for ICD-10 are not available (as of January 2006).

Pharmacokinetic data

The pk family of commands is aimed at analyzing pharmacokinetic data, especially at assessing bioequivalence; see [R] **pk**.

Survey data

The `svy` family of commands accounts for the sample design in survey studies. Facilities include adjustment for sampling weights, clustering, and stratification. You can find an introduction in [U] **26.16 Survey data** and more detail in the *Survey Data Reference Manual*. See a brief example in section 13.4.

Time-series data

Stata has several commands for analyzing time series data, which are described in the *Time-Series Reference Manual*.

Panel data

Panel data reflect repeated measurements on individuals or other study objects. Such data have a time structure, and they are clustered in the sense that the measurements on an individual are not independent. The `xt` family of commands is used for analysis; it is described in the *Longitudinal/Panel Data Reference Manual*. See a brief example in section 13.4.

17 Advanced topics

This chapter discusses several advanced Stata facilities. You may find it useful if you have basic experience and feel a need to go beyond the basics. The chapter is not intended to replace the general manuals, and if you are a bit ambitious, you need the *Programming Manual* as well.

17.1 Using saved results

Many Stata commands leave information behind at termination, called *saved results*. Commands such as predict and rvfplot (section 13.1), stphplot and estat phtest (section 14.3), lincom (chapter 13 and section 15.4), and lroc (section 15.4) are *postestimation* commands; they use information (saved results) left by other commands at completion. For an overview, see [U] **20 Estimation and postestimation commands**. For most estimation commands, the *Reference Manual* includes a section on postestimation commands, e.g., [R] **logistic postestimation**.

Many users would never wish to know more than this, but if you do, read more about saved results in [U] **18.8 Accessing results calculated by other programs**. If you want to know even more, read [R] **estimates**, [P] **return**, and [P] **ereturn**.

Commands are e-class, r-class, or n-class; n-class commands, such as generate, do not save results. We start with the simplest: r-class commands.

Saved results from r-class commands

summarize is an r-class command; it saves results in r(). After we run summarize, the command return list displays the names and contents of the saved results:

```
. cd C:\docs\ishr
. use ras.dta, clear
(Diagnosis of renal artery stenosis)
. summarize crea
```

Variable	Obs	Mean	Std. Dev.	Min	Max
crea	437	93.12815	24.45286	51	189

```
. return list
scalars:
                  r(N) =  437
              r(sum_w) =  437
               r(mean) =  93.12814645308924
                r(Var) =  597.9422564188693
                 r(sd) =  24.45285783745674
                r(min) =  51
                r(max) =  189
                r(sum) =  40697
```

One `summarize` command can analyze many variables; the saved results refer to the last variable. The saved results can be used by other commands; here `display` calculates the standard error from the standard deviation (`r(sd)`) and the number of valid observations (`r(N)`). `quietly` suppresses the output from `summarize`, but the results are still saved:

```
. quietly summarize crea
. display "Standard Error = " r(sd)/sqrt(r(N))
Standard Error = 1.1697388
```

The saved results are not part of the dataset but can be considered temporary constants that are available for analysis. They exist until they for some reason disappear, such as when you run another r-class command.

Saved results from e-class commands

Regression analysis commands and several other commands are estimation or e-class commands; they save results in `e()`. Here we use `logistic` as an example. To see the saved results from an e-class command, use `ereturn list`:

```
. use ras.dta, clear
(Diagnosis of renal artery stenosis)

. logistic stenosis renogram crea
```

Logistic regression   Number of obs   =   437
                                                 LR chi2(2)   =   152.91
                                                 Prob > chi2   =   0.0000
Log likelihood = -158.59076   Pseudo R2   =   0.3253

stenosis	Odds Ratio	Std. Err.	z	P>|z|	[95% Conf. Interval]	
renogram	17.68998	5.228973	9.72	0.000	9.911079	31.57429
crea	1.017621	.005813	3.06	0.002	1.006291	1.029078

```
. ereturn list
scalars:
                    e(N) =  437
                 e(ll_0) = -235.0458401292179
                   e(ll) = -158.5907608452163
                 e(df_m) =  2
                 e(chi2) =  152.9101585680031
                 e(r2_p) =  .325277312893391
               e(N_cdf) =  0
               e(N_cds) =  0

macros:
                  e(cmd) : "logistic"
              e(predict) : "logistic_p"
                e(title) : "Logistic regression"
               e(depvar) : "stenosis"
             e(crittype) : "log likelihood"
           e(properties) : "b V"
            e(estat_cmd) : "logit_estat"
             e(chi2type) : "LR"

matrices:
                    e(b) :  1 x 3
                    e(V) :  3 x 3
                e(rules) :  1 x 4

functions:
                e(sample)
```

Find a description of these saved elements in [R] **logistic**.

Postestimation commands such as lincom (see sections 13.1, 13.2, and 15.4) use the results saved in e(). If you get the error message last estimates not found, it means that the results needed are not available for some reason, and we must run logistic again; here we do it quietly to avoid displaying the output again:

```
. lincom renogram + 70*crea + _cons
last estimates not found
r(301);
. quietly logistic stenosis renogram crea
. lincom renogram + 70*crea + _cons
 ( 1)  renogram + 70 crea + _cons = 0
```

stenosis	Odds Ratio	Std. Err.	z	P>|z|	[95% Conf. Interval]	
(1)	1.167837	.3299007	0.55	0.583	.671317	2.031595

lincom itself is an r-class command; it saves in r():

```
. return list
scalars:
                  r(se) =  .3299007364313011
            r(estimate) =  1.167837393719094
```

Information saved in c()

These are not really results, but you can see several Stata settings and constants by typing

```
. creturn list
```

One of the constants displayed is π:

```
...
c(pi) = 3.141592653589793
...
```

The statsby command

`statsby` (see [D] **statsby**) collects saved results from a command, and it may be done across a by list.

Using the `lbw1.dta` dataset, we want to create a graph displaying the estimated mean birthweight with confidence intervals for three racial groups. We could obtain the coordinates with

```
. by race, sort: ci bwt
```

and you could enter them with an `input` command, as in the do-file generating figure 11.32.

`statsby` uses the results saved after a command, but first we must know their names:

```
. use lbw1.dta, clear
(Hosmer & Lemeshow data)

. ci bwt

    Variable |      Obs      Mean    Std. Err.    [95% Conf. Interval]
-------------+-------------------------------------------------------
         bwt |      189   2944.286    53.02811     2839.679    3048.892

. return list

scalars:
              r(ub) =  3048.892293354518
              r(lb) =  2839.67913521691
              r(se) =  53.02811244558399
            r(mean) =  2944.285714285714
               r(N) =  189
```

If we are in doubt about the meaning, we can look up the appropriate manual entry; here it is obvious that we are interested in `r(mean)`, `r(ub)` (upper 95% confidence limit), and `r(lb)` (lower confidence limit).

We can now create a new dataset containing three observations, one for each race, and four variables: race, mean birthweight, and lower and upper confidence limits:

```
. statsby mean=r(mean) cil=r(lb) ciu=r(ub), by(race) clear: ci bwt
(output omitted)

. list
```

	race	mean	cil	ciu
1.	1. white	3103.01	2955.53	3250.491
2.	2. black	2719.692	2461.722	2977.662
3.	3. other	2804.015	2628.076	2979.954

statsby is a prefix command, like by and xi; here it is a prefix to the ci bwt command that followed the colon. r(mean), etc., are the results saved by ci bwt. The clear option allows us to overwrite the current dataset.

Overwriting the current dataset can be avoided by the saving() option, as in the following do-file that generates figure 17.1:

```
                          ──── gph_fig17_1.do ────
* gph_fig17_1.do

cd C:\docs\ishr
use lbw1.dta, clear


statsby mean=r(mean) cil=r(lb) ciu=r(ub), ///
  by(race) saving(bwtrace.dta, replace): ci bwt

use bwtrace.dta, clear
set scheme lean1

twoway                                 ///
  (scatter mean race)                  ///
  (rcap cil ciu race)                  ///
  ,                                    ///
  xtitle("Race")                       ///
  ytitle("Birthweight, grams")         ///
  xscale(range(0.5 3.5))               ///
  xlabel(1 2 3, valuelabel notick)     ///
  legend(off)                          ///
  xsize(3) ysize(2.2) scale(1.4)
```

(Continued on next page)

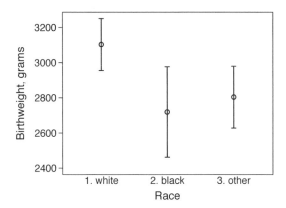

Figure 17.1: `statsby` used to generate coordinates (mean, 95% CI) for a graph

Figure 11.32 was created by entering data from a `summarize` output into a do-file with an `input` command. The coordinates can, however, be generated directly from the original data, as shown in the do-file `gph_fig11_32b.do`, which is available at this book's web site. The data management in this case was quite complex because several variables were involved.

17.2 Macros

You can read more about macros in [U] **18.3 Macros** and [P] **macro**.

A Stata macro is a kind of variable that has a *name* and *contents*. The content is a character string, but the string may represent a numeric value. A macro is not part of a dataset, but the information is available to the current program or session. In a command including a macro name, the name is replaced by the content before execution; this replacement is called *macro expansion*.

Stata's use of the word *macro* differs from another common usage. *Cambridge Advanced Learner's Dictionary* defines a macro as a "single instruction given to a computer which produces a set of instructions for the computer to perform a particular piece of work". In Stata terminology, this is more like the definition of a program, and Stata macros could have been given the name *micro*.

Local macros live within a program or a session, but only as long as the program or the session is active. Global macros (not to be discussed further here) are those that can be accessed by other programs.

Local macros are typically defined by the `local` command. When used as arguments to other commands, they are put in single quotes, such as 'SE'. The left single quote is ' (accent grave); the right quote is the simple ' (apostrophe).

> **Hint: Producing the left single quote:** In this book, the appearance of single quotes differs a bit from how they look on your keyboard and screen. Try `help quotes` to see how they look on the screen. Keyboard layouts differ, and on some keyboards, the left single quote is produced by a dead key, meaning that nothing is produced until you hit the spacebar.

I chose—although this is not standard—to use capital letters for macro names to distinguish them clearly from variable names.

In section 17.1, we saw the following construct after `summarize`:

```
. quietly summarize crea
. display "Standard Error = " r(sd)/sqrt(r(N))
Standard Error = 1.1697388
```

Now, if we want to use the standard error, e.g., for calculating a confidence interval, we must somehow store it. Storing it as a variable in the dataset is not economical; it would mean storing as many copies as there are observations. Instead we store the mean and standard error as the local macros `MEAN` and `SE` and use them to calculate confidence limits:

```
. quietly summarize crea
. local SE = r(sd)/sqrt(r(N))
. local MEAN = r(mean)
. display "Mean = " 'MEAN' "  SE = " 'SE'
Mean = 93.128146   SE = 1.1697388
. local CIL = 'MEAN' - 1.96*'SE'
. local CIU = 'MEAN' + 1.96*'SE'
. display "95% CI: " 'CIL' " - " 'CIU'
95% CI: 90.835458 - 95.420835
```

Before execution of the command

```
. local CIL = 'MEAN' - 1.96*'SE'
```

the macro names are replaced by the macro contents. After expansion, the command is

```
. local CIL = 93.128146 - 1.96*1.1697388
```

The macros above contained numerical information. We can also define a local macro directly as a string, without an equal sign:

```
. local VLIST "stenosis renogram crea"
```

The content of VLIST is the string "stenosis renogram crea". Before execution, the command

```
. logistic 'VLIST'
```

expands to

```
. logistic stenosis renogram crea
```

This macro could be useful if you are going to perform several analyses using the same list of variables.

There is a third form of macro definition: extended functions, which use a colon after the macro name; you can read more in [U] **18.3.6 Extended macro functions**. In the following example, the `variable label` macro function copies the content of the variable label associated with the variable v1 to the macro content:

```
. local LBL : variable label v1
```

At the end of section 17.3, under *Debugging programs*, is an illustration of macro expansion.

17.3   Programs

This section shows how you can write your own small programs or commands as ado-files. An ado-file is much like a do-file, but you execute it by calling its name, possibly followed by one or more arguments. The first significant line is a `program` command, and the last is an `end`. The filename must correspond to the name in the `program` command.

To work, an ado-file must be placed in an *ado-path* folder; see section 1.1. Your *ado-path* folder names are displayed by `sysdir`. The folder for your personal creations typically is `C:\ado\personal`, and we will use that in the following discussion.

Imagine that you repeatedly find yourself issuing `list` commands with the `clean`, `nolabel`, and `noobs` options (see section 10.2). Actually, you often forget the options and get frustrated. You can tailor your own command for such listings, e.g., calling it `mylist`. (First, do a `findit mylist` to make sure that the name does not conflict with existing official or unofficial commands). The simplest possible ado-file would be this `mylist.ado`:

```
—————————————————————— mylist.ado ——————————
program mylist                    // version 1
list, clean noobs nolabel
end
```

Issuing this `mylist` command will make a list of all variables in all observations, applying the `clean`, `nolabel`, and `noobs` options, and you might want more control. `syntax` helps you; see [U] **18.4.4 Parsing standard Stata syntax** and [P] **syntax**. A better version of the program is

```
—————————————————————— mylist.ado ——————————
program mylist                    // version 2
syntax [varlist] [if] [in]
list 'varlist' 'if' 'in', clean noobs nolabel
end
```

Now the command

```
. mylist mpg-weight if price>10000
```

does exactly the same as the command

```
. list mpg-weight if price>10000, clean noobs nolabel
```

This simple example illustrates a strong feature of Stata: you can generate your own commands.

lprob.ado estimates the probability of an outcome

In section 15.4, we used `adjust` after `logistic` to estimate the probability of stenosis, given information on the renography result and the serum creatinine level. We could have used `adjust` again, but for illustrative purposes, we will instead use `lincom`:

```
. cd C:\docs\ishr
. use ras.dta, clear
(Diagnosis of renal artery stenosis)
. quietly logistic stenosis renogram crea
. lincom renogram + 70*crea + _cons
 ( 1)  renogram + 70 crea + _cons = 0
```

stenosis	Odds Ratio	Std. Err.	z	P>|z|	[95% Conf. Interval]	
(1)	1.167837	.3299007	0.55	0.583	.671317	2.031595

Remember that the result of `lincom` depends on the results saved by the preceding estimation command; any independent variables included in the `logistic` command, but not in the `lincom` command, are still included—with the value 0. Had we, after the `logistic` command above, written `lincom _cons + renogram`, we would get the odds for stenosis among hypothetical patients with an abnormal renography and a serum creatinine level of 0.

When including _cons in the arguments for `lincom` after `logistic`, the coefficient is an odds, not an odds ratio as indicated in the heading. To get the corresponding probability, we type

```
. display 1.167837/2.167837
.53871071
```

If we need to enter this sequence repeatedly, would it not be nice to have a command displaying the probability directly? It certainly would be safer. (Actually, `adjust` does that for you, but for now we pretend that it does not.) To illustrate the idea, I created the `lprob1` command to be used after `logistic`; it gives the probability of the outcome with 95% confidence interval. We do not need to specify _cons; it is included automatically.

```
. lprob1 renogram + 70*crea

( 1)   renogram + 70 crea + _cons = 0
```

stenosis	Odds Ratio	Std. Err.	z	P>|z|	[95% Conf. Interval]
(1)	1.167837	.3299007	0.55	0.583	.671317 2.031595

```
Probability: .53871079      95% CI: .40166702 - .67014287
```

We did this by creating the ado-file C:\ado\personal\lprob1.ado. The first command in an ado-file is program followed by the program name; the program name must match the name of the ado-file. The last command is end:

```
──────────────── C:\ado\personal\lprob1.ado ────────────────
program lprob1

lincom '0' + _cons
local LN_0 = ln(r(estimate))
local SE_LN_0 = r(se)/r(estimate)
local CIL = exp('LN_0' - 1.96*'SE_LN_0')
local CIU = exp('LN_0' + 1.96*'SE_LN_0')
local PROB = r(estimate)/(1+r(estimate))
local CIL = 'CIL'/(1 + 'CIL')
local CIU = 'CIU'/(1 + 'CIU')
display " "
display " Probability: " 'PROB' "      95% CI: " 'CIL' " - " 'CIU'

end
```

The information available from lincom is the odds for stenosis (r(estimate)) and the standard error for odds (r(se)). To calculate a confidence interval, we need ln(odds) and SE(ln(odds)); the latter can be calculated by SE(odds)/odds. (The standard error displayed by lincom is actually calculated as SE(ln(odds))*odds, so we reverse this calculation.) From ln(odds) and SE(ln(odds)) you can calculate the confidence limits for ln(odds), and from here things are straightforward.

In the second command in the above program (lincom '0' + _cons), the 0 (zero) is a local macro name; it contains whatever was input after the command name; here it was renogram + 70*crea. The macro name is put in single quotes, meaning that it will be replaced by its contents before execution; after expansion, the command is

```
. lincom renogram + 70*crea + _cons
```

Now we create the local macro LN_0; it contains the result of the expression ln(r(estimate)), i.e., ln(odds).

r(se) is another saved result from lincom: the standard error of the estimate. We calculate SE(ln(odds)) and assign the result to the local macro SE_LN_0.

The contents of local macro CIL is the lower 95% confidence limit for the odds—same procedure for the upper limit.

Let local macro PROB contain the probability: odds/(1+odds). Replace the values in CIL and CIU in the same way.

Here is the final version of the lprob program; it creates output like this:

```
. lprob renogram + 70*crea

Probability of stenosis (Stenosis at angiography):
0.538711 (95% CI: 0.401669 - 0.670141)
```

This version of lprob.ado includes comments and aims at to be fail-safe:

```
                          ──────── C:\ado\personal\lprob.ado ──────────
*! lprob ver 1.0 27apr2005
*! Calculates probability of outcome after -logistic- or -logit-.
*! Author: Svend Juul
  program lprob
  version 9


* Check that we have saved results from -logistic- or -logit-
  if "`e(cmd)'" != "logistic" & "`e(cmd)'" != "logit" {
     display as error "lprob only works after -logistic- or -logit-"
     error 301
  }


* If no arguments, include _cons.
* If _cons is specified, don't include it again;
* otherwise include it.
  if "`0'" == "" {                              // No arguments
     quietly lincom _cons, or
  }
  else if strpos("`0'","_cons") {              // _cons specified
     quietly lincom `0', or
  }
  else {                                        // None of the above
     quietly lincom `0' + _cons, or
  }

  local LN_0 = ln(r(estimate))                 // ln(odds)
  local SE_LN_0 = r(se)/r(estimate)            // SE(ln(odds))

* Instead of 1.96, use the more precise invnormal(0.975)
  local CIL = exp(`LN_0' - invnormal(0.975)*`SE_LN_0')  // CI for odds
  local CIU = exp(`LN_0' + invnormal(0.975)*`SE_LN_0')  // CI for odds
  local PROB = r(estimate)/(1 + r(estimate))            // Probability
  local CIL = `CIL'/(1 + `CIL')                         // CI for probability
  local CIU = `CIU'/(1 + `CIU')                         // CI for probability
```

```
* We want the dependent variable's label in output.
  local VARLAB : variable label `e(depvar)'

* If the dependent variable has no label, don't try to include it;
* if it has, include it in parenthesis.
  display " "

  if "`VARLAB'" == "" {                              // No variable label
     display as result "Probability of `e(depvar)':"
  }
  else {                                             // Variable label
     display as result "Probability of `e(depvar)' (`VARLAB'):"
  }

  display as result ///
     %08.6f `PROB' " (95% CI: " %08.6f `CIL' " - " %08.6f `CIU' ")"

end
```

If an ado-file is of more permanent value—especially if it might be used by others—it should have a header with a short description. If you want quick information about a command, use the `which` command:

```
. which lprob

C:\ado\personal\lprob.ado
*! lprob ver 1.0 27apr2005
*! Calculates probability of outcome after -logistic- or -logit-.
*! Author: Svend Juul
```

This program has been tested with Stata version 9, and if you try to run it with version 8, it might malfunction. `version 9` will therefore give an error message if you try it with version 8. In future Stata versions, some functionalities might change, but typing `version 9` ensures that the program will still be working. The rest of the program is probably self-explanatory.

Having created a program that might be useful to others, you may want to make it public at the SSC archives; see section 2.2. You also must create a help-file; see [U] **18.11.6 Writing online help**.

After I developed the `lprob` program, I discovered that the `adjust` command does what I wanted. I decided, however, to keep the description of `lprob` to illustrate the development of an ado-file. Like `lincom`, `adjust` is a postestimation command. Running it after a `logistic` command with the `pr` and `ci` options, we get the following:

```
. quietly logistic stenosis renogram crea

. adjust renogram=1 crea=70, pr ci
```

```
Dependent variable: stenosis     Command: logistic
Covariates set to value: renogram = 1, crea = 70
```

All	pr	lb	ub
	.538711	[.401669	.670141]

```
Key:  pr       = Probability
      [lb , ub] = [95% Confidence Interval]
```

Debugging programs

If a program is interrupted by an error message, we cannot see which program line created the error. We might also have a program that does not give the result intended. Example: a previous version of lprob was lprob2:

```
———————————— C:\ado\personal\lprob2.ado ————————
program lprob2

lincom '0' + _cons
local LN_0 = ln(r(estimate))
local SE_LN_0 = r(se)/r(estimate)
local CIL = exp('LN_0' - 1.96*'SE_LN_0')
local CIU = exp('LN_0' + 1.96*'SE_LN_0')
local PROB = r(estimate)/(1+r(estimate))
local CIL = 'CIL'/(1 + 'CIL')
local CIU = 'CIU'/(1 + 'CIU')
display " "
display " Probability: " 'PROB' "     95% CI: " 'CIL' " - " 'CIU'

end
```

Running it gives the following output:

```
. lprob2 renogram + 70*crea
 ( 1)   renogram + 70 crea + _cons = 0
```

stenosis	Odds Ratio	Std. Err.	z	P>|z|	[95% Conf. Interval]	
(1)	1.167837	.3299007	0.55	0.583	.671317	2.031595

```
96* invalid name
r(198);
```

I had difficulty locating the error. However, with

```
. set trace on
```

all program lines will be displayed, including other programs called by the program. The amount of output may be overwhelming, but you can restrict it by typing

```
. set tracedepth 1
```

Comparing the expanded commands with your expectations can give you a clue:

```
. set trace on
. set tracedepth 1
. lprob2 renogram + 70*crea
```

                                                                  ── begin lprob ──
```
- lincom '0' + _cons
= lincom renogram + 70*crea + _cons

 ( 1)   renogram + 70 crea + _cons = 0
```

stenosis	Odds Ratio	Std. Err.	z	P>|z|	[95% Conf. Interval]
(1)	1.167837	.3299007	0.55	0.583	.671317 2.031595

```
- local LN_O = ln(r(estimate))
- local SE_LN_O = r(se)/r(estimate)
- local CIL = exp('LN_O' - 1.96*'SE_LN_O')
= local CIL = exp(.1551536570080954 - 1.96*)
96* invalid name
```

```
r(198);
```
                                                                  ── end lprob ──

For lines including a macro, you first see the original program line, preceded by −, and next the expanded command, preceded by =:

```
- lincom '0' + _cons
= lincom renogram + 70*crea + _cons
```

Looking at

```
- local CIL = exp('LN_O' - 1.96*'SE_LN_O')
= local CIL = exp(.1551536570080954 - 1.96*)
96* invalid name
```

you discover that 'SE_LN_O' expanded to nothing. This is a common mistake: the macro name should be SE_LN_O (capital O), but I had written SE_LN_0 (zero). Now let's correct the error. Remember we need to set trace off before proceeding. Read more about debugging in [P] **trace**.

17.4   Useful programming commands

The term *programming commands* does not mean that the commands can be used only in programs, i.e., ado-files; they can be used in do-files, as well, and even interactively. The following commands are documented in [P] *Programming Manual.*

if ... else if ... else

Do not confuse the `if` *command* with the `if` *qualifier* (section 4.4). The `if` *qualifier* asks questions to the data for each observation (`... if crea < 70`), and this leads to selection of the observations to be processed. The `if` *command* asks questions of the command environment, e.g., about the contents of a certain macro, and this leads to selecting commands to be used on all observations, as in

```
if "`0'" == "" {                         // No arguments specified
   quietly lincom _cons, or
}
else if strpos("`0'","_cons") {          // _cons specified
   quietly lincom `0', or
}
else {                                   // None of the above
   quietly lincom `0' + _cons, or
}
```

The meaning of the `else if` and `else` commands should be obvious. The braces must be used exactly as shown: the opening brace, {, comes at the end of the command, and the closing brace, }, on a line of its own. The purpose of the indentation is to improve legibility; it means nothing to Stata. When there is only one command between the braces, you can omit them, and you thus could have written the above construct as

```
if "`0'" == ""               quietly lincom _cons, or
else if strpos("`0'","_cons") quietly lincom `0', or
else                         quietly lincom `0' + _cons, or
```

foreach

Section 10.3 demonstrates a shortcoming of `tab2`: if we want cross-tabulation of one variable with several other variables, we must give as many commands as we want tables. Here we want a crosstable of each of the variables q1-q10 with `treat`. The `foreach` command solves the problem:

```
foreach Q of varlist q1-q10 {
   tab2 `Q' treat
}
```

The local macro `Q` is a stand-in for q1 to q10, and the construct generates 10 commands:

```
tab2 q1 treat
tab2 q2 treat
...
```

`foreach` commands can be nested, and you could create a cross table for each of the variables r1-r5 with each of the variables c1-c10 (a total of 50 tables):

```
foreach R of varlist r1-r5 {
   foreach C of varlist c1-c10 {
      tab2 'R' 'C'
   }
}
```

Although foreach is described in the *Programming Manual*, it can be used as an ordinary command in do-files as well, and even interactively. Here we interactively create 5 observations with five variables containing random numbers between 0 and 1. You enter these six lines in the Command window or in a do-file:

```
clear
set obs 5
foreach Q of newlist q1-q5 {
   generate 'Q' = uniform()
}
list
```

In the output, it looks like this, with the commands numbered within the foreach loop:

```
. clear
. set obs 5
obs was 0, now 5
. foreach Q of newlist q1-q5 {
  2.     generate 'Q' = uniform()
  3. }
. list
```

	q1	q2	q3	q4	q5
1.	.0264971	.8116255	.0522238	.1895829	.9307174
2.	.1727387	.1745866	.349758	.0624414	.3240527
3.	.0292306	.2453097	.5232757	.1508073	.4708069
4.	.7537692	.1119462	.3259046	.577387	.3824427
5.	.6555921	.7595286	.2854945	.958726	.6267027

The rules for the placement of braces are the same as for if. foreach takes different types of lists; read more in [P] **foreach** or help foreach. Above you saw varlist referring to existing variables and newlist referring to variables to be created. numlist refers to a number list; see the example in the next section (forvalues).

forvalues

forvalues lets you loop over a numeric range. The following trivial example illustrates the principle:

```
. forvalues I = 1/3 {
  2.      display 'I'
  3. }
1
2
3
```

The numeric range may be specified as shown, or as, e.g., (0(5)25), but not all numeric list forms (see section 4.3) are allowed; see [P] **forvalues** or help forvalues. If you want to loop over the values 4, 3, 2, 7, 6, 5, 4, 3, 2, 1, a standard numeric list could be 4/2 7/1, but forvalues will give an error message:

```
. forvalues I = 4/2 7/1 {
  2.      display 'I'
  3. }
invalid syntax
r(198);
```

You can solve this problem by using foreach with numlist, which accepts standard numeric lists, such as

```
. foreach I of numlist 4/2 7/1 {
  2.      display 'I'
  3. }
4
3
2
7
   (output omitted)
```

Parallel lists

If you have experience from Stata version 7 and earlier, you might recall the for command, which has been removed in favor of foreach and forvalues. One of the nice things, however, was the ability to handle parallel lists. Below I show how this can be obtained by using forvalues; see a cute FAQ (http://www.stata.com/support/faqs/lang/parallel.html) and a paper by Cox (2003a).

We have the variables x1-x5 and y1-y5, and we want to generate the variables z1-z5, where z1=x1*y1, z2=x2*y2, etc. The values of the primary variables are

```
. list
```

	x1	x2	x3	x4	x5	y1	y2	y3	y4	y5
1.	0	8	1	2	9	9	10	7	7	4
2.	2	2	3	1	3	1	0	0	5	5
3.	0	2	5	2	5	1	4	10	1	6
4.	8	1	3	6	4	5	3	7	9	0
5.	7	8	3	10	6	1	6	3	1	0

With `forvalues`, we can do the following:

```
. forvalues I=1/5 {              // I takes the values 1,2,3,4,5
  2.     gen z`I' = x`I' * y`I'  // z-variables are the products:
  3. }                          // z1=x1*y1, z2=x2*y2, etc.
. list
```

	x1	x2	x3	x4	x5	y1	y2	y3	y4	y5	z1	z2	z3	z4	z5
1.	0	8	1	2	9	9	10	7	7	4	0	80	7	14	36
2.	2	2	3	1	3	1	0	0	5	5	2	0	0	5	15
3.	0	2	5	2	5	1	4	10	1	6	0	8	50	2	30
4.	8	1	3	6	4	5	3	7	9	0	40	3	21	54	0
5.	7	8	3	10	6	1	6	3	1	0	7	48	9	10	0

Here the structure of variable names made the solution rather simple, but what if the variables are a-e and p-t and we want to generate the variables ap=a*p, bq=b*q, etc.? The primary variables are

```
. list
```

	a	b	c	d	e	p	q	r	s	t
1.	0	8	1	2	9	9	10	7	7	4
2.	2	2	3	1	3	1	0	0	5	5
3.	0	2	5	2	5	1	4	10	1	6
4.	8	1	3	6	4	5	3	7	9	0
5.	7	8	3	10	6	1	6	3	1	0

The trick is to use `describe` with the `simple` option (see [D] **describe**). It saves a list of variable names in `r(varlist)`, and the lists are assigned to the local macros XVARS and YVARS:

```
. quietly describe a-e, simple  // list variable names a-e to r(varlist)
. local XVARS "`r(varlist)'"    // local macro XVARS contains variable names
. quietly describe p-t, simple  // list variable names p-t to r(varlist)
. local YVARS "`r(varlist)'"    // local macro YVARS contains variable names
```

Next take the pairs of variables to be multiplied, using the extended macro function `word`
... of to pick variables sequentially (see [U] **18.3.6 Extended macro functions**):

```
. forvalues I=1/5 {                    // I takes the values 1,2,3,4,5
  2. local X : word `I' of `XVARS'   // Assign the Ith word of "a b c d e" to
                                        //     macro X
  3. local Y : word `I' of `YVARS'   // Assign the Ith word of "p q r s t" to
                                        //     macro Y
  4.     gen `X'`Y' = `X' * `Y'      // variable XY is the product of two
                                        //     variables:
  5. }                               // ap=a*p, bq=b*q, etc.
```

```
. list
```

	a	b	c	d	e	p	q	r	s	t	ap	bq	cr	ds	et
1.	0	8	1	2	9	9	10	7	7	4	0	80	7	14	36
2.	2	2	3	1	3	1	0	0	5	5	2	0	0	5	15
3.	0	2	5	2	5	1	4	10	1	6	0	8	50	2	30
4.	8	1	3	6	4	5	3	7	9	0	40	3	21	54	0
5.	7	8	3	10	6	1	6	3	1	0	7	48	9	10	0

Other commands

continue within a foreach or forvalues loop returns control to the foreach or forvalues command, thus skipping the remaining commands in the current loop iteration. continue, break jumps to the next command after the loop. See [P] **continue** for more information on continue.

```
forvalues I = 1/1000 {
   if 'I' > 100 {
      continue, break
   }
   display 'I' "   " sqrt('I')
}
```

capture can be used in do-files and ado-files to allow the job to continue despite an erroneous command; the standard behavior is that the job is terminated. It can be used, for example, to generate specific error messages (although this one is not that specific). _rc is an error code that reflects the error status of the last command; it is 0 if the command is valid. See [P] **capture** for more information about capture.

```
capture summarize var1
if _rc != 0 {
   display as error "Variable does not exist"
}
```

17.5   Do-files and ado-files useful for handling output

Elaborate profile.do

In chapter 1, you saw a simple profile.do, which automatically opens an output log file (stata.log) and a command log file (cmdlog.txt) at the start of a session. Here is a more elaborate version that adds a time stamp to the command log file, which will make it easier for you to reconstruct previous work. profile.do puts the log files in C:\ (the root folder), but of course you may decide to put them elsewhere.

The time stamp is created using the c-class date and time macros. You may include a DOS command by prefixing it by `shell` or `!`; see [D] **shell**.

```
─────────────────── C:\ado\personal\profile.do ───────────────────
* C:\ado\personal\profile.do  executes automatically when opening Stata.

* Write session start time in time.txt.
  set obs 2
  gen time="******* Session started: `c(current_date)' `c(current_time)'"
  replace time=" " if _n==1
  outfile time using "C:\time.txt", noquote replace
  clear

* Copy session start time to the cmdlog (cmdlog.txt) and open it.
* ! means that a DOS command follows.
  ! copy  /b  C:\cmdlog.txt + C:\time.txt  C:\cmdlog.txt  /y
  cmdlog using "C:\cmdlog.txt", append

* Open the output log in text format (stata.log)
* for display in a text editor or the Viewer.
  log using "C:\stata.log", replace

* If you want an output log in smcl format (stata.smcl)
* for display in the Viewer, replace the above line with:
*    log using "C:\stata.smcl", replace
```

Ado-files for handling output

If you have an active output log, *Ctrl-L* lets you view it in the Viewer or suspend or close it. This method will work regardless of the name and type (text or SMCL) of your output log.

Your output log may have become large, so you want to start a fresh log. The `newlog` command lets you do that. The content of a minimal `newlog.ado` is

```
─────────────────── C:\ado\personal\newlog.ado ───────────────────
program newlog
log close
log using C:\stata.log, replace
end
```

The above ado-file will work, but it can be improved:

```
────────────────────────── C:\ado\personal\newlog.ado ──────────────────────────
*! newlog ver 1.0 30jul2005
*! Closes current output log and opens a new output log.
*! Author: Svend Juul

program define newlog
version 9
args LOG
if "'LOG'" != "" {
  capture log close
  log using "'LOG'", replace
}
else {
  quietly log
  local LOG "'r(filename)'"
  if "'LOG'" == "" {
    log using C:\stata.log, replace
  }
  else {
    log close
    log using "'LOG'", replace
  }
}

end
```

newlog may be called with a log filename, in which case the current log, if any, is closed
and a new log with the specified filename opens:

    . newlog mylog.log

If you call newlog without a filename it examines whether a log is open, in which case it
is replaced by a new log with the same name. Otherwise, the text output log C:\stata.log is
opened.

I prefer using a general text editor to inspect and modify output before printing; compared
with using the Viewer window, you have more freedom, and you can use the keyboard instead of the mouse to edit. This method requires a text output log. My favorite text editor,
NoteTab Light, can be downloaded for free; you can find a short description and a link to its
web site at the author's web site. See *Other supplementary materials provided by the author* at
http://www.stata-press.com/books/ishr.html. nlog opens a copy of the output log in NoteTab
Light. The content of nlog.ado is

```
————————————— C:\ado\personal\nlog.ado ——————————
*! nlog ver 1.0 27apr2005
*! Opens output log in NoteTab Light
*! Author: Svend Juul

program nlog
version 9
quietly log

if "'r(filename)'" == "" {
   display as error "No log file"
}
else {
   winexec "C:\Program files\NoteTab Light\NoteTab.exe" "'r(filename'"
}

end
```

The Stata command winexec executes a Windows command. Obviously, you need to check where NoteTab Light was installed and modify nlog.ado accordingly.

If you let profile.do open a command log at the start of a program, you can inspect it in the Do-file Editor using the ecmd command. The content of ecmd.ado is

```
————————————— C:\ado\personal\ecmd.ado ——————————
*! ecmd ver 1.0 13feb2005
*! Opens command log in a Do-file editor window
*! Author: Svend Juul

program ecmd
version 9
quietly cmdlog

if "'r(filename)'" == "" {
   display as error "No command log file"
}

else {
   copy "'r(filename)'"  "C:\_cmd.log", replace
   doedit "C:\_cmd.log"
}

end
```

In `profile.do`, I used the `append` option to preserve commands issued at previous sessions. However, the Do-file Editor's capacity is limited, and you must now and then delete the command log.

The above `profile.do` and ado-files are available at this book's web site, http://www.stata-press.com/books/ishr.html. Download them to `C:\ado\personal` if you want to use them.

18 Taking good care of your data

The purpose of this chapter is to give some preventive advice: how to protect yourself against mistakes, errors, loss of data, and wasted time. Avoiding these pitfalls requires you to work systematically and pay consistent attention to documentation issues. A more elaborate version of this chapter can be found in the web book *Take Good Care of Your Data* (Juul 2005); see *Other supplementary materials provided by the author* at http://www.stata-press.com/books/ishr.html.

I have seen quite a few accidents with data—including some where I had only myself to blame—that could have been prevented with modest investments in documentation and safeguards. These were accidents such as

- Not being able to reconstruct a published result.

- Not being able to explain why the number of participants in the dataset was 157; it ought to have been 159.

- Having trouble understanding your own data when you return to them after a 4-week break.

- Making a mistake on how data were coded, thus arriving at an erroneous result.

- Working on the wrong dataset.

- Not being able to restore archived data (they were on a tape that no existing tape drive can read).

- Having taken careful backup—and storing the backup media in the same room as the computer (the office burned).

Such incidents at least lead to wasted time; sometimes the consequences are much worse. But prevention is not that difficult.

18.1 The audit trail

When keeping financial accounts, such as for a company or an association, there are some obvious principles to follow:

It must be possible to go back from the balance sheet to the individual vouchers. This is done by giving each voucher a unique number. From each item in the balance sheet, you must be able to identify the component amounts and the corresponding vouchers. The term *audit trail* means exactly this: from the final results you must be able to follow the trail backward to the primary sources of information. If you are the bookkeeper, you need this for yourself; otherwise, you will have a hard time tracing errors. And it is mandatory for auditing.

The same principles apply when handling information in research. You should be able to trace each piece of information back to the original source document:

- ID (case identifier) must be included in the original documents and in the dataset.
- All corrections must be documented and explained.
- All modifications to the dataset must be documented by do-files.
- All major analyses must be documented by do-files.

This technique is needed during error checking and correction, when generating new variables, and when your project is exposed to external audit and monitoring.

The purposes are primarily to protect yourself against mistakes, errors, waste of time, and loss of information, secondarily to enable external audit. Documentation procedures must be included during project planning, and they should be with you all the time.

18.2   Data collection

The design of your data collection instruments like questionnaires and case report forms can have strong implications for the quality of your data. For some advice, see Juul (2005). You might search the net using keywords such as "questionnaire layout" to find more advice; I found one I liked from University of Leeds at http://www.leeds.ac.uk/iss/documentation/top/top2.pdf.

With questionnaires, there are two important considerations:

1. The respondent: the questionnaire should be designed to minimize the risk of mistakes and errors.
2. The data processing: the questionnaire should be easy to handle, and the risk of coding and transcription errors should be minimized.

The first consideration is by far the most important; there is no way to correct a respondent's mistakes afterward.

Collect and record raw, not processed, information

Avoid grouping continuous information at data collection time. It is as easy for the respondent to state her age in years as to choose between age groups. Even better: the date of birth allows you to let the computer calculate the exact age at any other time.

18.3   The codebook

The codebook is the link between the original data and the data entered in the computer, and it should be prepared early in the process. Here is a short example:

Variable	Source	Meaning	Codes, valid range	Format[a]
id	Q1	Questionnaire number	1–750	3.0
sex	Q2	Respondent's sex	1 Male 2 Female 9 No response	1.0
byear	Q3	Year of birth	1890–1990 -2^b No response	4.0
schooled	Q4	Left school, level	1 Before finishing 9th 2 After 9th 3 After 10th 4 After high school 5 Other 9 No response	1.0
children	Q5	No. of children	0–10 -2^b No response	2.0
voced	Q6	Vocational education	1 None 2 Manual, <3 years 3 Manual, 3 years + 4 Nonmanual, <3 years 5 Nonmanual, 3–4 years 6 Nonmanual, 5 years + 7 Cannot be classified 9 No response	1.0

[a] This notation is often used when describing formats. 2.0 means a numerical variable with two digits and no decimals. 5.2 means five digits, including a decimal period and two decimals. A 10 means a 10-character string (text) variable. You might use Stata's format descriptors instead, such as %3.0f.

[b] Missing values for interval scale variables should not be included in calculations.

Codes

Standard recommendation: always use numerical codes. Not all analyses can handle string codes (e.g., "M" for male sex), and numerical codes are faster to enter and easier to handle during analysis. For interval-scale variables (year of birth, number of children), just use the value as the code, and state the possible range in the codebook. For categorical variables (sex, education), state the meaning of each code. This information should be included in the dataset as value labels.

For open questions, the text information should not be entered as is in the computer, but you must translate the text into a finite number of categories; they should be described in the codebook. Add a coding field next to the response field, and design it so that it does not confuse respondents. Before deciding on a final classification, you might want to classify a sample of, for example, 100 responses to see if it works.

People do not always fill in questionnaires as you expect. You asked about cups of coffee per day and expected a single number, but you got responses like "2–3" and "2–4". For such situations devise a rule, such as "Calculate the average, and round up if necessary".

The codes for missing values require special attention; see section 5.3.

18.4   Folders and filenames: the log book

Sections 18.5–18.7 illustrate the steps from data entry to a final dataset for analysis. In your own research, there may be more steps, so there is good reason to plan ahead. Here is some advice on decisions that should be taken early.

Choose which folder to use for the project

My strong advice is to organize your folders by subject, not by file type. For a specific project or subproject, keep all your main text files, data files, and do-files in the same folder; an illustration is shown in appendix B. Do not mix files from different projects in the same folder. Take a copy of the final data and do-files, and put them in a "safe" folder.

Never put your own files in a program folder. You may never find them again, or they may be destroyed if you upgrade the program.

Decide a system for naming your data and do-files

Do-files that add modifications to your data are vital documentation. It is tempting to issue single commands, one at a time, but it is a lot safer to create a do-file with all commands needed and execute them together—in the right sequence. You will make errors while developing a do-file, but in the end you will succeed, and you should, of course, keep only the correct do-files for documentation. The vital do-files should include everything needed—but nothing else—to reconstruct the data from the original input.

These do-files should have names clearly indicating what they do. I offer the suggestion to let such do-files start with gen_, followed by the name of the result file. Do-files that do not create new versions of the data should *not* have this prefix. Other systems may be used, but without a system you risk confusion. The log book illustrates my suggestion for naming the data and do-files used in sections 18.6–18.7.

Choose a system for variable names

If you have only a few variables, use names that give intuitive meaning, as in the codebook section 18.3. If you have a lot of variables, instead use names derived from, e.g., question numbers: q7a, q7b, etc.; an intuitive system will break down for you. In complex projects where you have data from several sources, use variable names that reflect the source. If you have three interviews with the same persons, use the prefixes a, b, c:

1st interview: a1 a2 a3a a3b a3c etc.

2nd interview: b1 b2 etc.

Keep a log book—and keep it updated

To review your past actions, keep a log book and update it whenever you add modifications to your data. This log book corresponds to the data modifications performed in sections 18.6–18.7.

Project: Treatment of diseaseX			
Working folder: C:\docs\disx			
Safe folder: C:\docs\disx\safe			
Input data	Do-file	Output data	Comments
visit1a2.rec visit1a.rec (EpiData files)	exported from EpiData	visit1a.dta	12 oct 2004 Final comparison of two corrected data entry files. Agreement documented in visit1_compare.txt
visit1a.dta	gen_visit1b.do	visit1b.dta	13 oct 2004 Add labels to visit1a.dta
visit1b.dta	gen_visit1c.do	visit1c.dta	15 oct 2004 Identified errors corrected (see visit1_correct.doc)
visit1c.dta visit2c.dta	gen_visit12.do	visit12.dta	16 oct 2004 Merging data from visit 1 and visit 2
visit12.dta	gen_visit12a.do	visit12a.dta	16 oct 2004 Generate new variables: hrqol, opagr

Make a master do-file

I recommend making a master do-file corresponding to the log book; this file is just a series of do commands that ensure that you perform tasks in the right sequence. Imagine that you discovered an error when analyzing data. You could now incorporate the correction in `gen_visit1c.do` and from the master do-file run that and the subsequent do-files again:

```
─────────── master.do ───────────
* master.do
cd C:\docs\disx
* Add labels
do gen_visit1b.do
* Correct errors
do gen_visit1c.do
* Merge data from visit 1 and visit 2
do gen_visit12.do
* Generate new variables
do gen visit12a.do
```

Instead of using the `cd` command, we could have defined the full path for each file. The important thing is to define the path, one way or the other:

```
─────────── master.do ───────────
* master.do
* Add labels
do C:\docs\disx\gen\_visit1b.do
* Correct errors
do C:\docs\disx\gen\_visit1c.do
* Merge data from visit 1 and visit 2
do C:\docs\disx\gen\_visit12.do
* Generate new variables
do C:\docs\disx\gen\_visit12a.do
```

18.5   Entering data

With small datasets, we can enter data in Stata's Data Editor, but with larger datasets this method is cumbersome and error prone. Instead, use a data entry program such as EpiData; see section 6.2. You can also find a short description and a link to its web site from the author's web site; see *Other supplementary materials provided by the author* at
http://www.stata-press.com/books/ishr.html. EpiData can be downloaded for free.

Preparations

Before entering data, you need to have a complete codebook. All decisions on coding should be made—and documented in the codebook—before you enter data; otherwise the risk of errors increases.

Examine the source documents (e.g., questionnaires) for obvious inconsistencies before you enter data. Do any coding of text information before, not during, data entry, and write it in the source document.

When defining the dataset, you need the codebook information on variable names and formats (the number of digits needed to represent the information).

Especially when you have data from several sources, you need to write down a plan for the process, including the folder structure, file names, and variable names. Also make a plan on how to back up your work to reduce the consequences of human, software, or hardware errors; see section 18.9.

Error prevention

A good data entry program such as EpiData enables you to create forms resembling your questionnaire or case report form pages; this reduces the risk of misplacing information during data entry. "Parallel shifting" during data entry is a common source of error: a correct value is entered, but in the wrong place.

If you enter the wrong ID number, it may be hard to locate and correct the error. I suggest that you reenter the ID number as the last field in the data entry form as a safeguard.

EpiData lets you specify valid values and value labels for each variable; you then get a warning during data entry if you enter an outlier. While this method identifies illegal values, it does not catch erroneous entries within the legal range. You may also specify extended checks, for example, that a date of hospital admission is after the date of birth. However, specifying the rules correctly may be time-consuming, and incorrect specifications will interfere with data entry. Also, inconsistent responses—which can be quite frequent—can interfere with data entry. I prefer to check for illegal values later; see section 18.6.

EpiData lets you enter data twice (preferably by two different operators) and compare the contents of the two files to get a list of discrepancies. Examine the original source documents, and decide which entry was correct. Correct the errors in both files, and run a new comparison, which should show no errors. Keep this output as documentation that the dataset now is "clean".

Proofreading is a rather inefficient (and boring) way of error checking and is virtually impossible for large data volumes. At the least, you need an assistant and a printout of the data entered; proofreading data on the screen is inefficient and will strain your eyes.

Which level of safeguards should you use?

Use cost–benefit thinking. If you made a clinical trial with $50 + 50$ patients, the extra cost of double data entry is much lower than the total cost of collecting the information, and one error might affect the conclusion. You should do everything to avoid errors in your data. If, on the other hand, you mailed a questionnaire to 10,000 persons to estimate the prevalence of certain conditions, the consequence of one error is small, and you might decide to save the costs of double entry of every questionnaire.

Modern ways of entering data

Using optical reading is smart for large numbers of small questionnaires (such as the pools). For small numbers of large questionnaires, it is highly inefficient because of the time spent with preparations. The first consideration is to the respondent, but the layout requirements for optical reading may counteract this consideration.

Especially with telephone interviews, it might be practical to enter responses directly into the computer during the interview, thus avoiding the paper step. This is a good idea for simple mass surveys and opinion polls; however, for most research purposes, I discourage it, because setting up a correct form for data entry might be quite time-consuming, and if an unpredicted situation arises during an interview, you might get stuck. You will need a lot of experience to be able to do that.

18.6   Inspecting and correcting your data

With complex datasets, you should examine and make corrections to each partial dataset before merging files. In the following examples, there are two partial datasets: `visit1` and `visit2`.

Adding labels to your data

You should define variable and value labels (see section 7.1) in the codebook before you enter data, and you can let EpiData include them in the dataset before entering the data. You might, however, have received the raw data from another source. In that case, you should define labels now before examining the results. Stata does not need the labels, but *you* need them for readable output.

`gen_visit1b.do` is the do-file that generates the `visit1b.dta` dataset:

```
─────────────────────────── gen_visit1b.do ───────────────
* gen_visit1b.do generates visit1b.dta - 12 oct 2004
* Adding labels to primary data

cd C:\docs\disx
use visit1a.dta, clear

label variable id "Questionnaire number"
label variable sex "Sex of respondent"
label variable byear "Year of birth"
...
label define sexlbl  1 "male"  2 "female"
label values sex sexlbl
...
recode byear (9999=.a)
numlabel, add

save visit1b.dta, replace
```

This do-file includes vital documentation and should be saved and kept in a safe place. It starts with reading the input data file and ends with saving the modified dataset. I strongly recommend giving the do-file a name that tells what it does: `gen_visit1b.do` generates the `visit1b.dta` dataset. Include the do-file's own name as a comment in the first line.

The value 9999 was entered for missing year of birth; this code was recoded to Stata's user-defined missing code, `.a`. Stata does not display the codes and the value labels simultaneously in output, but the `numlabel` command incorporates the numeric codes in the value labels.

Searching for errors

Next, print a codebook, an overview of your variables, and simple frequency tables of appropriate variables:

```
. use visit1b.dta, clear
. describe
. codebook, compact
. label list occup
. tab1 sex nation-educ
. tab2 sex pregnant
```

`describe` and `codebook` give an overview of your variables. Look for the minimum, maximum, and number of valid values in the `codebook` output. `label list` shows value-label lists.

`tab1` shows tables for all variables mentioned (avoid tables for variables with many values).

`tab2` can disclose inconsistent information (such as pregnant males).

Since this job did not modify your data, you need not save the commands as a do-file for documentation. You may save it, but do not give it the `gen` prefix because it does not generate new data.

You *must* make a printout of the tables produced; do not use the screen. You can easily miss an error—and strain your eyes. Examine the following:

1. Compare the codebook created with your original codebook (section 18.3), and check that you made the label information correctly.
2. Inspect the overview table (`codebook, compact`), especially for illegal or improbable minimum and maximum values. Also check that the number of valid observations for each variable is as expected.
3. Inspect the frequency tables (`tab1`) for strange values and for values that should have labels but do not.
4. Examine tables that could indicate inconsistencies (such as pregnant males).

If you identified any suspicious values, list them with the ID number (which must also be written at the source document's front page), and control their correctness.

Data entry errors sometimes occur if you misplace the values entered. If you discover an error, also proofread the neighboring variables; they have a high risk of errors, as well. In the following commands, byear-diag represent sex and its neighbors; age1-educ represent pregnant and its neighbors:

```
. use visit1b.dta, clear
. list id byear-diag if sex>2, nolabel
. list id byear-diag age1-educ if sex==1 & pregnant==1, nolabel
```

Make a printout of the lists created; do not use the screen. Next go back to the original documents, identify the errors, and write the corrections on the lists. Examine the neighboring variables carefully; they are at high risk of error, as well.

Correction of errors

If you discover an error, you might intuitively go to the Data Editor and correct it there, but I discourage this method. First, the risk of "correcting" the wrong variable or observation is high. Second, the change will be poorly documented, breaking the audit trail.

You should make corrections in a do-file. The gen prefix indicates that this do-file generates a new version of the dataset.

```
────────────────────── gen_visit1c.do ──────────────────────
* gen_visit1c.do
* Corrections 14 oct 2004. See project log page 27.

cd C:\docs\disx
use visit1b.dta
replace sex=2 if id==2473
replace weight=75 if id==3771
...

save visit1c.dta
```

In this way, you have full documentation of the changes made to the dataset, and the audit trail is not broken.

On the other hand, if you discover errors when comparing files after double data entry, you can make corrections directly in the data entered, provided that you end this step with a new comparison of the corrected files and, it is hoped, demonstrating that there are no disagreements. The point is that you split the process in distinct and well-defined steps and that your documentation from one step to the next is consistent. But you should not bother documenting that you made and corrected errors during the data entry, any more than I should document which spelling errors I made and corrected while writing the text in front of you.

Handling inconsistent information

Data may have been entered correctly, but the respondent has filled in the questionnaire inconsistently. A respondent might claim to be male and pregnant or to be 23 with her oldest son 19 years old.

Some researchers code all inconsistent data as missing, without further considerations. Others believe that the investigator should examine other information available and judge which piece of information is most likely to be correct. I recommend that the latter principle should be followed—with caution. But no matter which principle you follow, you will have made a decision on how to interpret data, and *such decisions must be documented in writing.*

The missing-data problem

A nonresponse is a nonresponse, but in certain cases, missing data have a high cost. In a regression analysis with 10 predictors, an observation is omitted from the analysis if just one predictor is missing. If many observations have one or more missing predictors, this leads to a heavy loss of information—and the result may be biased if nonresponse is related to one of the factors of interest.

There are formal remedies for this situation: one is missing-value imputation, where the most likely response is estimated from the characteristics of respondents with valid information; see [D] **impute**. There are some pitfalls to this solution, and the standard precondition of independence of observations is violated.

Sometimes you can make a reasonable judgment about missing data. For example, a woman whose children are 1, 9, and 20 years old is likely to be close to 40 herself. What is most correct, to consider her age unknown or to use 40 as a pretty close but imperfect judgment? If a respondent did not answer a question on a rare symptom, what is most correct, to treat it as no information or to consider it a "No"?

No matter what you decide, *you must document your decision in writing.*

Merging datasets

If you have several sources of data, make sure that all corrections have been made before merging; it is much more difficult to do afterward:

```
───────────────────────── gen_visit12.do ─────────────────────────
* gen_visit12.do
* Merge corrected visit1c and visit2c data sets.
cd C:\docs\disx
use visit1c.dta, clear
merge id using visit2c.dta, sort
save visit12.dta

tab1 _merge
list id _merge if _merge<3
```

Check that `merge` worked as intended (examine `_merge`; see section 9.5). Any unexpected mismatches might be due to errors in the matching variable (`id`) entered in one of the datasets, and such errors can be difficult to disentangle. Use the `duplicates report` command (see section 9.5) to check before merging whether the values of the matching variable are unique.

18.7   Modifying data

You should certainly not modify your original data, but you will often want to derive new variables from the original information. You might combine the information from several questions on well-being in one new variable or calculate the age from two dates and create 5-year age groups. When modifying data, follow these rules:

1. If you modify your data, the result should be saved as a file with a *new* name that indicates the version (include a, b, c or 1, 2, 3 in the filename).

2. The do-file containing the modifications must be saved with an appropriate name. I recommend using the gen prefix to illustrate that this do-file generates a new dataset.

3. The do-file must start with the command indicating the input data and end with the command indicating the output data. Commands that are not relevant to the modifications should be omitted from the do-file.

4. Include comments to explain (to yourself or others) the purpose of complex operations.

5. You can include further documentation in the dataset using the `label` and `note` commands.

gen_visit12a.do is the do-file generating `visit12a.dta`. It starts with the command reading the data (`use`) and ends with the command saving the modified data (`save`). Note the use of the `cd` command to make sure that the datasets are located as intended.

```
                         ─── gen_visit12a.do ───
* gen_visit12a.do
* generates visit12a.dta with new variables.

cd C:\docs\disx
use visit12.dta, clear


* Calculate hrqol: quality of life score.
egen hrqol=rowsum(q1-q10)
label variable hrqol "Quality of life score"

* Calculate opage: age at operation.
generate opage=(opdate-bdate)/365.25
label variable opage "Age at operation"

* Calculate opagr: age groups at operation.
recode opage (55/max=4 "55+")(35/55=3 "35-54")(15/35=2 "15-34") ///
   (min/15=1 "-14"), generate(opagr)
```

```
label variable opagr "Age at operation, 4 groups"

label data "Visit12a.dta created by gen_visit12a.do, 02 jan 2004"
save visit12a.dta, replace
```

Three new variables were created from the original information. To keep the original `opage` unchanged, I let the `recode` command generate the new variable `opagr`. You will want to define variable and value labels immediately after creating a new variable (you can do so within the `recode` command). It will never be easier than now, and it will make it much easier for you to read the do-file later.

Comments are helpful for explaining the purpose of complex operations.

`label data` attaches a label to the dataset to be displayed each time it is opened. Notes can be included in the dataset (`note`). You can display the notes included in a dataset by using the command `notes`; see section 7.1.

WARNING! Do not overwrite good data with bad data: use `save`'s `replace` option only if you really want to overwrite an existing dataset. Here it was justified because we made an error or omission in the first version of the do-file.

Check correctness of modifications

Errors do occur, and your modifications might not do what you intended. The modified do-file should demonstrate by your comments what you intended to do and by the commands what you actually did. Look at the distributions of the new variables, and list a sample of observations with both the source and target variables to check the correctness of calculations. By all means, print the lists before inspection! Reading on the screen is unreliable (and unpleasant, to say the least).

```
. use visit12a.dta, clear
. codebook hrqol opage opagr, compact
. tab1 opagr
. sample 1
. slist q1-q10 hrqol
. sort opage
. list bdate opdate opage opagr
```

In the `codebook` output, look for the number of valid observations and for minimum and maximum values. `tab1` is useful for variables with few categories, like `opagr`. The last commands are performed on a 1% sample only. `slist` lets you compare `hrqol` with the original values of `q1-q10` and the derived age variables with the original dates. (`slist` works better than `list` with many variables; you can find and download it with `findit slist`; see section 10.2.) Sorting by `opage` makes the comparisons between `opage` and `opagr` easier.

If you identify inconsistencies you must go back, modify gen_visit12a.do, and check again.

18.8   Analysis

Make sure you use the right dataset

For analyses beyond the simplest, I recommend using do-files, starting with the command that reads the data. There are two reasons for this recommendation:

1. You might during a session have made temporary modifications to your data (e.g., a selection of cases, or recoding a variable)—and forgot that you did that.

2. Documenting an analysis includes documenting which dataset you used.

```
──────────────────────────── regress_sbp.do ────────────────────────────
* regress_sbp.do

cd C:\docs\disx
use visit12a.dta, clear

regress sbp sex
regress sbp sex weight
regress sbp sex weight height
predict psbp
rvfplot, yline(0)
lincom _cons + 1*sex + 175*height + 80*weight
```

Late discovery of errors and inconsistencies

Despite your efforts to secure data quality, you may during analysis discover errors and inconsistencies. It is an obvious advantage to correct all errors before analysis, but if you organized your do-files, corrections are not that difficult: go back and modify the correction do-file (gen_visit1c.do, section 18.6). Run this and the subsequent do-files, and you have a corrected analysis file. If you followed the recommendations in section 18.4 (log book, naming of do-files, a master do-file), this is easy. If not, the procedure will be time consuming and error prone.

18.9   Backing up and archiving

The distinction between backing up and archiving may seem subtle, but the purposes are different. *Backing up* is an everyday activity, and its purpose is to allow you to restore your data and documents in case of destruction or loss of data. Destruction may be physical, but most cases of data loss are due to human errors, such as unintentional deletion or overwriting of files.

Archiving takes place once or a few times during the life of a project. The purpose is to preserve your data and documents for a more distant future, maybe even to allow other researchers access to the information.

The computer professionals I know are trustworthy people, but their occupational mobility is high. Ask your supervisor or department if there is a local policy on issues of data protection, ownership of data, and responsibility for proper managing, backing up, and archiving data. Unfortunately in many departments, these issues are not as clearly stated as they should be—in writing. If the department has no written instructions, take the full responsibility yourself. If there are instructions, evaluate them and decide if you need any further safeguards.

Backing up data

Strategy considerations

The way you handle your own data greatly affects your ability to back up and restore your data. I will especially point to the following issues:

- Using a logical and transparent folder structure is good for your everyday work—and makes it easier to back up and recover your data. Appendix B suggests a folder structure where your own data and documents are kept separately from program folders: all of your "own" files are located in subfolders under your main folder (C:\docs in this book).

- Back up not only datasets but also do-files modifying your data and written documents: protocol, codebook, log book, and other documenting information.

By far the safest strategy is to regularly back up all of your files using a semiautomated procedure; see below.

Do a *full backup* with regular intervals, e.g., every 6 months. This backup includes all of your data and documents—but not program files.

Take an *incremental backup* regularly, e.g., at the end of each working day. Include all new files and any files modified since the last backup.

Filenames are important. I recommend that you give your backup files names that enable you to sort them by age: 200512191723.zip for a zip file created at 5:23 P.M. on 19 December 2005. If you need to restore your data, start with the oldest to avoid overwriting new files with older versions.

Software considerations

There are several software options to consider. A good compression program is useful for backing up—and for other purposes, as well. I created the bkup command, which makes an incremental or full backup from a folder of your choice (e.g., C:\docs), including subfolders, to a compressed zip file with the name structure shown above. You can download bkup from this book's web site. It requires that the WinZip compression program be installed on your computer; you can read more in the accompanying help file (help bkup).

Media considerations

It is important that you store your backup media in a building other than the one where your computer resides; in case of fire you may otherwise lose all data.

Diskettes are cheap but not very stable. If you rely on diskettes, you should make two copies to be stored separately.

*CD-ROM*s and *DVD*s are quite stable, provided careful storage, but the experience with long-term stability is limited.

Magnetic tape is probably history by now. Stability varies.

Sending to a remote computer is my main recommendation; it requires no hardware beyond an Internet connection. If you have access to a server (located in a different building) you might use it for storing your backup files. Or you might have a mutual agreement with a friend living elsewhere to exchange backup files by email. Security and privacy considerations might lead you to encrypt the backup files; see later in this section.

Test your backup copy

Make sure that you actually can restore the data from your backup. If you use diskettes, CDs, or tapes, you must test them on a *different* computer, as the drives on other computers may differ in calibration.

Archiving

What to archive?

Whereas backing up is an everyday activity, archiving takes place once or a few times during the life of a project. If you worked with your data using consistent documentation procedures, archiving is easy. If not, it is difficult. The final archiving of a project should include the following:

- Study protocol.
- Applications to and permissions from ethical review boards, etc.
- Data-collection instruments (e.g., questionnaires, case-report forms).
- Coding instructions and other technical descriptions.
- The log book (see section 18.4) and other written documentation on the processing of data.
- At least the first and the final version of your data.
- All do-files that modify data. The do-files should enable reconstruction of the final version from the first version of your data.
- Publications.

Where?

Archiving research data should be institutionalized, either by a research institution or a public or private agency. Opportunities vary, but there is an increasing understanding of the need for such an institution. The opportunities in Denmark are an excellent model.

The Danish State Archives has a division for storing electronic information, Danish Data Archive (http://www.dda.dk), which offers safe archiving of research data at no cost. The level of access is determined by the investigator, who can decide that she only has access herself, that others can get access with her permission, or that the data are accessible to anybody. The major Danish research funds request that data be archived at Danish Data Archive at the end of a project.

If you are affiliated with a research institution, it should take responsibility for archiving of data—ask for written guidelines. However, many health researchers do not have a stable affiliation with a research institution, and that increases the need for some central organization.

Archiving data and keeping them readable is an active process where data are transformed to media and kept in formats that are still readable. In my department's basement, we until recently stored 8" and 5 1/4" floppy disks, magnetic tapes in various sizes, and even boxes with punch cards. To read them, we would probably need the help of a technical museum.

When?

There is no point in archiving undocumented data. Remember that archiving means storing for future use—in contrast to backup, which ensures viability of data in the short term. But waiting until completion and publication of the study can give you trouble; at that time, it can be difficult to collect the documents describing the process and to remember the computers on which the different versions of the data and do-files are kept.

The appropriate time for archiving depends on the project, but in general a two-step strategy is advisable:

1. Archive the raw dataset when you have finished entering data, corrected errors, and documented the data (see sections 18.6–18.7). Include all important documents, and archive copies of both data and the do-files that document modifications to data.

2. After analysis, archive updated data files and the corresponding do-files. Include copies of publications and other major documents written since the last archiving.

Isn't it difficult?

Archiving need not be difficult. If you have worked consistently with your data, you just need to archive the first and last datasets and the do-files documenting the modifications. If not, archiving is difficult—perhaps impossible.

18.10   Protecting against abuse

Motives and opportunities

Obviously sensitive information about people must be kept confidential without giving other persons the opportunity to see the information.

The *motives* for intruding could be curiosity (my neighbor's mystery disease), economic gain (should we insure Mr. NN?), creation of newspaper headlines ("Researchers fool around with confidential data"), and other indecent motives (if it becomes known that XX handles his data carelessly he will get in trouble—and I would love that).

It is the obligation of the researcher to give no other person the *opportunity* to see confidential information. Below I show two key methods to prevent unauthorized access to confidential electronic information.

Securing the electronic information is not enough; information on paper must also be protected against unauthorized access. Information on paper is more vulnerable to accidental access than the information in a computer file.

Remove external identifiers

To link the source documents (e.g., questionnaires) with the dataset, you usually give each person a unique number also to be recorded in the dataset. This number is an internal identifier that has no meaning outside your project, as opposed to external identifiers (name, social security number). While analyzing, you usually do not need to keep any external identifiers in the dataset, so you should remove them.

Removing an external identifier is simple:

```
                        ── gen_safe_keyfile.do ──
* gen_safe_keyfile.do removes external identifier

cd C:\docs\disx
use unsafe.dta, clear
keep intid extid
save a:\keyfile.dta

use unsafe.dta, clear
drop extid
save safe.dta


* When you have made sure that both files are valid:
erase unsafe.dta
```

The key file (`keyfile.dta`) linking the internal identifier (`intid`) with the external identifier (`extid`) should be encrypted and stored separately, i.e., not on the same computer as the information. It might be a good idea to store the key file at an archiving facility. Here I used a diskette, but beware that diskettes are not very stable, so make an extra backup copy.

If you later need to include `extid`, such as for matching with external data:

```
————————————— gen_unsafe.do —————————————
* gen_unsafe.do adds external identifier to data

cd C:\docs\disx
use safe.dta, clear
sort intid
merge intid using a:\keyfile.dta, sort

save unsafe.dta
```

Encryption

There are several possibilities for encryption; I use the WinZip compression program, at the same time saving disk space. It is easy and fast—but of course, you must neither forget your encryption password nor enable others to read it.

A Manuals and other good books

A.1 Stata manuals

The complete set of manuals comprises 17 volumes, but most users can make do with less. Here I list them with the manuals most relevant to health researchers first—although this list could be made in several ways. You can see more information about the manuals at http://www.stata.com/bookstore/.

[GS] *Getting Started.* There are separate manuals based on the operating system, [GSW] for Windows, [GSM] for Macintosh, and [GSU] for Unix.

[I] *Quick Reference and Index.* This book will help you find your way through the documentation.

[U] *User's Guide* gives a systematic overview and description of the Stata language, as well as many useful hints.

[D] *Data Management Reference Manual.* Includes all commands relevant to calculation and other data management commands. The content roughly matches chapters 8 and 9 of this book.

[R] *Base Reference Manual.* This three-volume manual includes the bulk of Stata commands, except those in [D] and some other specialized commands that are described in the manuals listed below.

[G] *Graphics Reference Manual.* Describes the commands to produce graphs.

[ST] *Survival Analysis and Epidemiological Tables Reference Manual.* The main part of this manual is devoted to survival analysis. Also, some other analyses frequently used in epidemiology (Mantel–Haenszel analysis) are included. The content roughly matches chapters 12 and 14 of this book.

[TS] *Time-Series Reference Manual.* Includes commands and other tools for time-series analysis.

[XT] *Longitudinal/Panel Data Reference Manual.* Analysis of repeated measurements, as in panel studies.

[SVY] *Survey Data Reference Manual.* Analysis of complex survey data. Includes discussions of poststratification, linearization, balanced repeated replication, and jackknife variance estimation methods.

[MV]   *Multivariate Statistics Reference Manual.* Includes several multivariate tech-
       niques, such as cluster analysis, factor analysis, principal components analysis,
       and correspondence analysis.

[P]   *Programming Reference Manual.* Includes several commands typically used in
       programs (ado-files).

[M]   *Mata Reference Manual.* A systematic description of the matrix programming
       language, Mata, introduced with the version 9 release of Stata.

A.2   Other books on Stata

An increasing number of books on Stata and books using Stata to illustrate epidemiological and
biostatistical methods are being published. The best place to look for books on Stata is Stata's
own bookstore at http://www.stata.com/bookstore/. Take a look now and then for new titles and
new editions of existing books.

I have no intent to assess each of the books listed below, and I selected books of specific
interest primarily to health researchers.

Hamilton, L. C. 2006. *Statistics with Stata. Updated for version 9.* Belmont, CA: Brooks/Cole.

Rabe-Hesketh, S. and B. Everitt. 2004. *A Handbook of Statistical Analysis Using Stata.* 3rd
       ed. Boca Raton, FL: Chapman & Hall/CRC.

Hills, M. and B. L. De Stavola. 2003. *A Short Introduction to Stata 8 for Biostatistics.* London:
       Timberlake Consultants Press.

Cleves, M., W. W. Gould, and R. Gutierrez. 2006. *An Introduction to Survival Analysis Using
       Stata.* 2nd rev. ed. College Station, TX: Stata Press.

Long, J. S. and J. Freese. 2006. *Regression Models for Categorical Dependent Variables Using
       Stata.* 2nd ed. College Station, TX: Stata Press.

Mitchell, M. 2004. *A Visual Guide to Stata Graphics.* College Station, TX: Stata Press.

A.3   Books using Stata

Several epidemiological and biostatistical textbooks use Stata more or less directly. Among my
favorites are

Kirkwood, B. R. and J. A. C. Sterne. 2003. *Essential Medical Statistics.* 2nd ed. Malden, MA:
       Blackwell Science.

       The book is pretty close in its priorities to this book. Stata commands and output are not
       presented directly, but the Stata datasets used are available at
       http://www.blackwellpublishing.com/essentialmedstats/datasets.htm.

Dupont, W. D. 2002. *Statistical Modeling for Biomedical Researchers.* Cambridge: Cambridge University Press.

The book includes many Stata examples, and the datasets used are available at http://www.mc.vanderbilt.edu/prevmed/wddtext/index.html#datasets.

Campbell, M. J. 2001. *Statistics at Square Two.* London: BMJ Books.

The analyses in the book were performed using Stata, and typical Stata output is presented.

B Advice on working with Windows

This appendix includes some tools and some advice on working with Windows. My main comments and recommendations apply to handling the folder (directory) structure. There are several ways to move and copy files; I show only one technique.

The techniques shown are a minimum of what you must be able to perform. Without them, you are at risk of creating accidents, either by losing important data or by being unable to locate them.

Create a smart folder structure

Do not mix your own data and documents with program files; to do so is risky and will inevitably lead to confusion. Create a personal main folder (the Documents folder), e.g., C:\docs, with all of your own files (data, do-files, text documents) in subfolders under the main folder. This approach will also facilitate backing up your data (see section 18.9). If you work in a networked setting, talk with your network administrator before restructuring things.

Your Windows installation may have placed your Documents folder somewhere along a long path under C:\Documents and Settings. This placement may complicate things to you, and I suggest (and in this book I assume in the examples) a simpler structure in which you make C:\docs your Documents folder.

First create the C:\docs folder (See *How to create a new folder*, later in this appendix).

Next make C:\docs your default main folder:

[Start] ▷ Settings ▷ Control Panel ▷ Administration

The appearance now depends on the Windows version you are using, but there should be an icon with the name Documents. Right-click it, and click Properties. Replace the current location of the default destination folder with C:\docs. When asked if you want to move folders and files from the current to the new location, answer Yes.

Organize your folder structure by subject, not by file type. Here is an example:

```
C:\
    ado
        personal
        plus
    docs
        ishr
        Personal
            CV
            Secrets (encrypted)
        Project 1
            Protocol
            Administration
            Data
                Safe
            Manuscripts
        Project 2
            Protocol
            Administration
            Data
                Safe
            Manuscripts
    Program files
        EpiData
        Games
            Solitaire
            GTA
        OpenOffice
        Stata9
            ado
                base
                updates
        WinZip
    Windows
```

This structure has several advantages, such as

- You avoid mixing your "own" files with program files.

- Your Documents folder (C:\docs) is the default root folder for all of your own subfolders (the white area), and when opening and saving files, you will look primarily at these folders, not the program folders.

- It is much easier to set up a consistent backup procedure (see section 18.9).

If your hard disk is partitioned into a C: and a D: drive, using C: for programs and D:\ as your Documents folder is a good idea:

```
C:\
      ado
          personal
          plus
      Program files
          ...
          Stata9
              ado
                  base
                  updates
          WinZip
      Windows
```

```
D:\
          ishr
          Personal
              CV
                  Secrets (encrypted)
          Project 1
              Protocol
              Administration
              Data
                  Safe
              Manuscripts
          Project2
          ...
```

How to select a default working folder for a program

The installation default working folder for many programs is the program folder itself. *This default is an extremely poor choice*, and you should never mix your own documents and data files with program files. You might never find your own files again; you might accidentally delete your data, such as when installing a new version of the program; or you might accidentally delete program files.

Stata initially suggests C:\data as the default working folder; this is a lot better, and it is okay when you are working with sample data. But as soon as you start working with real data, you should organize things by subject, not by programs. To define C:\docs as the default working folder for Stata, right-click the Stata desktop icon, and select

Properties ▷ Shortcut ▷ Start in   and then type C:\docs

Using Windows Explorer

I prefer using Explorer rather than My Computer. To put a shortcut at the desktop, find `explorer.exe` (typically in the `C:\Windows` folder). Right-click `explorer.exe`, drag it to the desktop, and select

> Create shortcut here

Make Windows display file name extensions

For reasons not understood by me, Microsoft decided not to display file name extensions by default. This choice is inconvenient (you cannot distinguish the do-file `alpha.do` from the dataset `alpha.dta`), so you should set Windows to display file name extensions. Open Windows Explorer, and select

> Tools ▷ Folder options ▷ View

You will see several check boxes. Uncheck Hide extensions for known file types.

Creating a new folder

Let's create a new folder: `project3` under `C:\docs`

- Double-click the Explorer icon at the desktop.
- Click `C:\docs` (root folder for own files).
- Select Files ▷ New ▷ Folder.
- Rename "`New Folder`" to "`project3`".

You can also use Stata's `mkdir` command (see section 6.1) to create a new folder:

```
. cd c:\docs
. mkdir "project3"
```

Renaming a folder or file

- In Explorer, right-click the folder or file and select Rename.
- Write the name desired, and press *Enter*.

Copying a file or a folder to another folder or to a diskette

- In Explorer, highlight the source file or folder; press *Ctrl-C* (copy to clipboard).
- Highlight the target folder (or `A:`); press *Ctrl-V* (paste from clipboard).

Stata's `copy` command performs the same functions (with some restrictions); see [D] **copy**.

How to move a file or a folder to another folder

- In Explorer, highlight the source file or folder icon, and press *Ctrl-X* (copy to clipboard and delete source file).

- Highlight the target folder and press *Ctrl-V* (paste from clipboard).

You may also copy or move files and folders using the mouse to drag and drop. But be aware that the effect is different whether you drag and drop within the same medium (disk) or between media. The *Ctrl-C*, *Ctrl-X*, *Ctrl-V* method works consistently, and it works much the same as when you are editing text in a word processor or in Stata's Do-file Editor.

Write-protecting a file

To prevent a file from accidental deletion or overwriting, you can write-protect it. To see the write-protection attribute for a file, right-click the file in Explorer, and select Properties. You can change the write-protection manually.

Smart users write-protect their vital data and do-files once they are satisfied with them.

References

Altman, D. G. 1991. *Practical Statistics for Medical Research.* London: Chapman & Hall.

Bland, J. M. 2000. *An Introduction to Medical Statistics.* Oxford: Oxford University Press.

Bland, J. M., and D. G. Altman. 1986. Statistical methods for assessing agreement between two methods of clinical measurement. *Lancet* I: 307–310.

———. 2003. Applying the right statistics: Analyses of measurement studies. *Ultrasound in Obstetrics and Gynecology* 22: 85–93.

Breslow, N. E., and N. E. Day. 1980. *Statistical Methods in Cancer Research, Volume 1.* 2nd ed. Lyon: IARC.

Campbell, M. J. 2001. *Statistics at Square Two.* London: BMJ Books.

Clayton, D., and M. Hills. 1993. *Statistical Models in Epidemiology.* Oxford: Oxford University Press.

Cleves, M., W. Gould, and R. Gutierrez. 2006. *An Introduction to Survival Analysis Using Stata.* 2nd rev. ed. College Station, TX: Stata Press.

Coviello, V., and M. Boggess. 2004. Cumulative incidence estimation in the presence of competing risks. *Stata Journal* 4: 103–112.

Cox, N. J. 2003a. Speaking Stata: Problems with lists. *Stata Journal* 3: 185–202.

———. 2003b. Speaking Stata: Problems with tables, Part II. *Stata Journal* 3: 420–439.

———. 2004. Speaking Stata: Graphing model diagnostics. *Stata Journal* 4: 449–475.

———. 2005. Some notes on text editors for Stata users. http://fmwww.bc.edu/repec/bocode/t/textEditors.html

Doll, R., and A. B. Hill. 1950. Smoking and carcinoma of the lung. Preliminary report. *British Medical Journal* 2: 84–93.

Dupont, W. D. 2002. *Statistical Modeling for Biomedical Researchers: A Simple Introduction to the Analysis of Complex Data.* Cambridge: Cambridge University Press.

Egger, M., G. Davey-Smith, and D. G. Altman. 2001. *Systematic Reviews in Health Care: Meta-Analysis in Context.* 2nd ed. London: BMJ Books.

Farley, T. M. M., M. M. Ali, and E. Slaymaker. 2001. Competing approaches to analysis of failure times with competing risks. *Statistics in Medicine* 20: 3601–3610.

Habbema, J. D., R. Eijkemans, P. Krijnen, and J. A. Knottnerus. 2002. Analysis of data on the accuracy of diagnostic tests. In *The Evidence Base of Clinical Diagnosis*, 117–144. London: BMJ Books.

Hosmer, D. W., Jr., and S. Lemeshow. 1999. *Applied Survival Analysis: Regression Modeling of Time to Event Data.* New York: Wiley.

———. 2000. *Applied Logistic Regression.* 2nd ed. New York: Wiley.

Juul, S. 2003. Lean mainstream schemes for Stata 8 graphics. *Stata Journal* 3: 295–301.

———. 2005. *Take Good Care of Your Data.* Aarhus: Institute of Public Health, University of Aarhus. http://www.folkesundhed.au.dk/uddannelse/software/takecare.pdf.

Kirkwood, B. R., and J. A. C. Sterne. 2003. *Essential Medical Statistics.* 2nd ed. Oxford: Blackwell Science.

Lindholt, J. S., S. Juul, H. Fasting, and E. W. Henneberg. 2005. Screening for abdominal aortic aneurysms: Single centre randomised controlled trial. *British Medical Journal* 330: 750–752.

Mitchell, M. 2004. *A Visual Guide to Stata Graphics.* College Station, TX: Stata Press.

Newson, R. 2004. Generalized power calculations for generalized linear models and more. *Stata Journal* 4: 379–401.

Pepe, M. S. 2003. *The Statistical Evaluation of Medical Tests for Classification and Prediction.* Oxford: Oxford University Press.

Pocock, S. J., T. C. Clayton, and D. G. Altman. 2002. Survival plots of time-to-event outcomes in clinical trials: good practice and pitfalls. *The Lancet* 359: 1686–1689.

Sackett, D. L., and R. B. Haynes. 2002. The architecture of dianostic research. In *The Evidence Base of Clinical Diagnosis*, ed. J. A. Knottnerus. London: BMJ Books.

Sackett, D. L., R. B. Haynes, G. H. Guyatt, and P. Tugwell. 1991. *Clinical Epidemiology. A Basic Science for Clinical Medicine.* 2nd ed. Boston: Little, Brown and Company.

Tukey, J. W. 1977. *Exploratory Data Analysis.* Reading, MA: Addison–Wesley.

University Group Diabetes Program. 1970. A study of the effects of hypoglycemic agents on vascular complications in patients with adult onset diabetes. *Diabetes* 19: 747–830.

Author index

Subject index